SELF-LOVE POTIONS

HERBAL RITUALS AND RECIPES
TO MAKE YOU FALL IN
LOVE WITH YOU

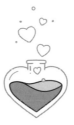

Cosmic Valeria

Illustrated by
Marie-Noël Dumont

CONTENTS

CHAPTER 3: HOME & BODY RITUALS

INTRODUCTION

This book was created in my garden and inspired by the recipes my mom taught me. I was born and raised in Siberia, a cold and harsh land where almost nothing blooms or flourishes. My parents moved there from Ukraine in search of a better life—they both grew up on farms, surrounded by plants and animals, and I remember how much they missed it. Every plant, every flower, every herb, every berry was cherished so much in our house. Not only because it was so hard to find them, but because we loved them so much. My mom taught me all about the properties of plants and how to preserve them. My dad taught me about forest magic and foraging. So, about five years ago, I started my very own garden. With no experience other than my parents' guidance, I nurtured plants from tiny seeds, elbow deep in dirt, and it has been the most rewarding and spiritual experience.

Plants not only provide us with an opportunity for self-care, they also keep us grounded and in the present moment. They inspire us to pay attention to the dirt under our feet, to the birds and worms; to get to know every single bush, tree, and flower of our neighborhood, as well as the forest around us. They serve as a reminder of our precious and limited time, and that it shouldn't be wasted on self-doubt or fear. Plants remind us to love, right here and now. To love unconditionally everything that surrounds us, and, most importantly, to love ourselves.

I hope this book inspires you to fall in love with plants and yourself over and over again. Thank you for allowing me to share this magic with you.

I love you,

Valeria

WHAT IS A SELF-LOVE POTION?

You have probably made a self-love potion or performed a magical ritual hundreds of times before without even realizing it. Intuitively choosing ingredients, setting intentions, perhaps lighting a candle. A love potion is not the number of crystals you put in your water or how many rose petals you add to your bath. A true self-love potion or ritual starts with a decision to carve some time out just for yourself, to heal your body and mind, to go deeper inward and find clarity, to make self-care and self-love a priority.

A self-love potion or ritual could be anything—a simple cup of tea or coffee in the morning, a quiet walk in the woods, a dip in the lake, the touch of a flower—so long as the intention is to love and treat yourself.

BEFORE WE GET STARTED

There is absolutely no wrong way to use this book. If you feel like adding another ingredient to a recipe, or changing a ritual, go for it! Your soul already knows what it needs, so don't resist it. Let this book be an opportunity for you to connect with your intuition and your inner knowledge; a reminder that everything you need and are looking for is already within. Pick a ritual or recipe that suits your intention and purpose, or simply open the book on a random page and see what the Universe has for you today.

- When it comes to kitchen rituals and casting spells, remember to source only flowers and herbs that have never been treated by pesticides or other harsh chemicals.

- Most edible flowers, spices, and roots are safe for us, but not for our four-legged friends. So keep all your kitchen magic away from pets.

- Many of the potions require minimal equipment, much of which you will already have in your kitchen. When anything more than this is required—such as storage jars, a journal for notes, or cheesecloth for straining—this is listed with the recipe.

- It is always a good idea to thoroughly clean and sterilize jars before making any potions. Sterilizing ensures that there are no harmful bacteria or residues left in the jar, prolonging the shelf life. The easiest way to do this is by simply boiling your jars. Place them in a large pot and fill it with water. Bring the water to a boil, and let it boil for at least 10 minutes.

Then carefully remove the jars from the pot—they are going to be very hot. As for the lids (plastic or metal), there is no need to boil them—simply wash them with warm, soapy water.

- Water rituals are incredibly relaxing, but take care when using oils, honey, and milk in the bath, because these items can make your bathtub extremely slippery. When cleaning your bathtub after taking a ritual bath, use a mesh strainer to scoop out all the ingredients (flowers, herbs, etc.) to avoid clogging the drain. Alternatively, you could use cloth/muslin bags when taking baths: simply put all the ingredients in the bag and place it under the warm running water to infuse your bath water, thus leaving no mess to clear up. Choose what works best for you. And if the opportunity presents itself, try to compost and return all the ingredients back to the earth. Always have a tall glass of water to hand in the bathroom, as hot baths can be very dehydrating.

- As for home and body rituals, try to be mindful and present in the moment as you perform them. Never leave incense burning or a candle unattended. And always remember to do a skin patch test for all homemade remedies (see page 118), especially if you have sensitive skin or are allergy-prone.

- Lastly, you don't have to consider yourself a witch to perform any of the spells or rituals in the book. Take what resonates with you and leave the rest.

A NOTE ON LOOKING AFTER YOURSELF

Herbal recipes can be very powerful and affective, but, as with many things, they can take time to work and may require some patience and perseverance to see results. It is also crucial to be aware and mindful of your body's unique needs, and to take care of yourself when using herbs on your body and in your home. You should consult with your doctor in any matters relating to your health, and you should not use the information in this book as a substitute for medication or other treatment prescribed by your medical practitioner.

Before trying any of the recipes in this book, please be aware of the following:

Some of these recipes suggest foraging for easily identified herbs. However, you should never ingest or touch a herb unless you are 100 percent certain of its identification, and it is always advisable to wear gloves whenever foraging because of the possibility of an allergic or other adverse reaction from the use of any flowers, herbs, or other plants mentioned in this book.

If you are pregnant, suffer from any allergies, or have any health concerns, seek advice from a medical herbalist or doctor before working with any herbs. If you feel unwell at any point or suspect you are having a reaction to a herb, seek medical advice immediately.

With herbal home cleaning product recipes, always apply to a small, inconspicuous area of furniture or surface first before applying to the whole thing. Even products that contain all natural ingredients can cause skin reactions in susceptible individuals. If you have sensitive skin that is prone to allergic reactions, wear gloves and apply the cleaning product in a well-ventilated area.

Keep any herbs away from pets and children, and take extra precaution when working with candles, or using oils in the bathtub.

Take care, look after yourself, and enjoy this book.

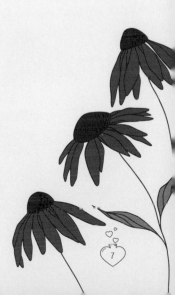

Self-love potions made in the kitchen are probably my favorite. Time spent in the kitchen is never wasted—it provides us with so many opportunities to be mindful and fully present, to feel and express gratitude, to nourish body and soul. But most importantly, the fragility and delicacy of plants reminds and inspires us to carve some time from our busy schedules and make self-care and self-love a priority.

Growing up, I watched my mom cook our meals with so much love and intention. She liked to stir the food clockwise, to promote and protect its energies. Before an exam or an important day at school, she would cook something with bay leaves, for good luck. And every time I would go on a class trip or leave for a summer camp, she would cook something warm and delicious with rosemary, for protection.

When it comes to magic, you can make your own rules. A kitchen spell could be anything you make in the kitchen. Plants infuse food with their magical properties—but of course, the main (and most important) ingredient is your intention. This is the starting point of every dream, every goal, every desire. Everything that happens in the Universe begins with it. Intention is a force, a strong purpose, an aim, a focus. And whatever you focus your energy on, you attract.

This chapter contains 28 easy-to-make love potions. Choose one that best suits your purpose, or pick one at random and see what the Universe has in store for you. When making potions in the kitchen or casting spells with your spatula, be fully present, set your intention in your head, or say it out loud. Don't try to rush the process, but rather admire and savor it. You are making magic with herbs and flowers, your kind words, and good thoughts—what could be more powerful than that?

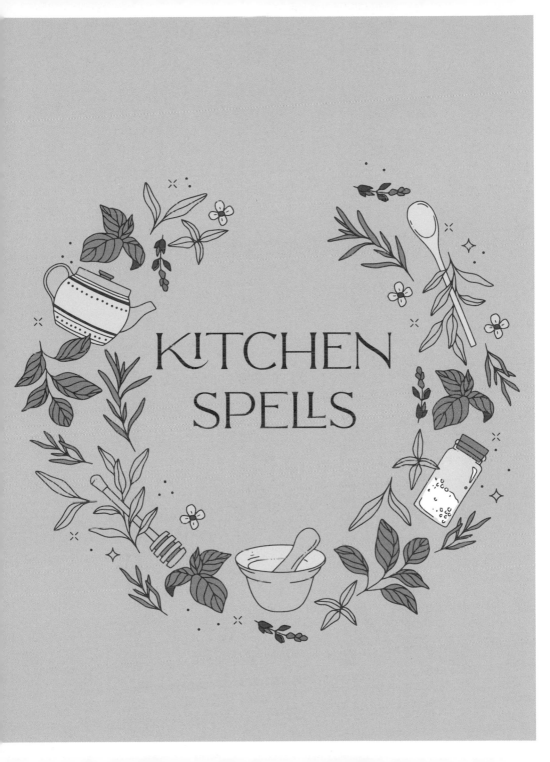

KITCHEN SPELLS

LILAC HONEY FOR INSPIRATION AND RENEWAL

There is a long history of witches using sugar, honey, maple syrup, and other sweeteners in their spells and rituals. The purpose of using a sweetener in a spell is to promote love, kindness, joy, and harmony while delivering what you truly desire: an easier, sweeter, more fluid life with fewer obstacles.

Lilac flowers bring us a sense of renewal, a new wave of inspiration. When we see the lilac flower, we know spring has arrived, and what a wonderful feeling that is. Traditionally, the flowers are associated with Easter, new beginnings and awakenings, and romantic relationships, and are believed to contain the essence of spring. Any time you need a little pick-me-up, a dose of inspiration and self-love, or simply want to bring excitement and sweetness into your everyday life, take a spoonful of this lilac potion.

In Eastern Europe lilac flowers are considered a symbol of wisdom and knowledge. Growing up, I remember families hovering lilac branches over their babies, to make them wise and smart. Other cultures consider lilac flowers a symbol of confidence, so lilac honey could be particularly supportive for someone about to embark on a new life adventure.

Ingredients:
½–¾ cup (16–24 g) fresh or dried organic lilac flowers
honey, as required

Equipment:
8 oz (225 ml) glass jar with lid

Directions:
Fill the jar three-quarters full with lilac flowers.

Pour the honey over the flowers, filling the jar almost to the top. Allow the honey to settle (this might take a while), then pour over any additional honey needed. The flowers will rise to the top.

Stir the honey every other day for the next two weeks.

Once the honey is infused, remove the lilac petals (simply scoop them off the top with a spoon) or leave them in for extra magic. They are 100 percent edible! Store the honey in your pantry for 2–3 months.

This infused, heart-soothing honey is delicious and can be used just like regular honey: spread it on toast, stir it into your tea or coffee, or add a few drops to a face mask.

BERGAMOT TEA
FOR SELF-ACCEPTANCE

Bergamot can be used for pretty much any magical ritual, from attracting abundance and luck, to cleansing and protecting your aura. But what bergamot is mostly known for is its ability to center you. It empowers you and lifts your spirit, so you can see that everything is perfect in this moment. And you are perfect too.

Bergamot is a wonderful plant to work with in times of uncertainty or insecurity. The delicate aroma awakens every cell in your body and reminds you of your own strength, which comes from a deep awareness of your divine nature and radical self-love and self-acceptance.

A simple cup of bergamot tea is a perfect example of how spells don't have to look a certain way, have a long list of ingredients, or be overly complicated in order to bring more magic and love into your everyday life.

Ingredients:
bergamot tea leaves
dash of honey or another sweetener (optional)
slice of lemon (optional)

Equipment:
candle (optional)
journal and pen

Directions:
Make yourself the most perfect cup of bergamot tea. Add sweeteners of your choice, and perhaps a slice of lemon.

Light your favorite candle to set the mood, if desired.

Grab your journal and pen and reflect on which areas of your life you have been denying love to yourself. How can you change that? What things are not in your control that you need to let go of? Are you holding yourself back because you can't accept and love every part of yourself? How can you change that? Are you allowing yourself to accept compliments from others? Are you complimenting yourself daily? If not, write at least ten compliments to your beautiful self. Remember, self-love always begins with self-acceptance.

We all go through times of doubting ourselves, feeling insecure, or lacking confidence. And it is ok to not feel ok sometimes. The key is to not let the negative thoughts ruin your day, month, or entire year. If a negative thought pops into your head, just be an observer. Allow the sensation to pass through your body. Acknowledge it and let it go. Not every thought or feeling needs to have a meaning.

FRIENDSHIP HEALING STRAWBERRY SALT

Friendships are just like any other relationship—they have their rough patches from time to time and occasionally require some work. I am sure I am not alone when I say I have lost many friends over the years—to distance and time, or to new interests. And that is ok, it is part of life. But there are other instances when I regret not doing more to save a friendship, or when I don't think I was that good a friend myself.

If you are looking to make new friends or want to heal your current friendships, try this dazzling strawberry salt. Strawberries symbolize the sweetness of life, and the joy of simple things. And strawberry salt is a great example of how two opposites can come together in a perfect and balanced union. This salty treat is meant to be shared and enjoyed with a friend—sprinkle it on your favorite dessert, or make a sugar rim for your cocktails (it's especially good with margaritas). Let it be another reason to connect and spend quality time with your friends.

Ingredients:
2 oz (55 g) freeze-dried strawberries
2 oz (55 g) kosher or coarse sea salt

Directions:
Start by grinding the freeze-dried strawberries in a food processor.

In a bowl, combine the strawberries with the salt (the suggested ratio is 1:1).

Pour and enjoy, or store in a cool, dry place in a container with a tight-fitting lid. Use within one week.

As children, friendships seem so easy and effortless. Just living in the same neighborhood brings you together. So at what age do we begin questioning our friends? Or ask for more from them? Try this potion to get your friendships back on track.

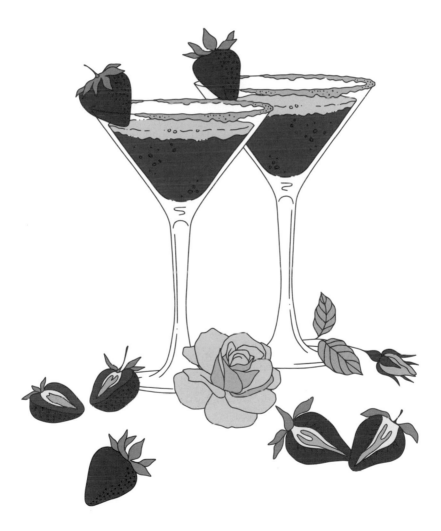

NASTURTIUM PESTO FOR MANIFESTATION

Bright nasturtium blooms are flowers you fall in love with at first sight. Associated with strength, purity, and strong emotion, nasturtium is believed to help balance emotions and rational thinking. High in vitamin C, and with antibacterial, antifungal, and antiseptic qualities, it is a perfect companion plant and always attracts pollinators.

Nasturtium is also destined to be worshipped in the kitchen. The leaves, flowers, and even the seeds are edible, delicious, and spicy. It is perfect for salads and garnishes, and the larger leaves are excellent for stuffing. My favorite dish is nasturtium pesto—because if making your own pasta sauce from scratch using flowers isn't an act of self-love, I don't know what is.

Some say that the nasturtium is for intellectuals, whose excessive thinking depletes their life force. It is also believed to symbolize the urge to fight for what one believes in, including patriotism. This is possibly because the shape of the flower looks a lot like a combat helmet.

Ingredients:
1 cup (40 g) nasturtium leaves and flowers
1 cup (25 g) basil leaves
2 tbsp pine nuts (you could also use walnuts, cashew nuts, almonds, or sunflower seeds)
2 tbsp freshly squeezed lemon juice
2–3 garlic cloves, to taste
½ cup (45 g) freshly grated Parmesan cheese (optional)
½ cup (120 ml) olive oil
salt and freshly ground black pepper

Equipment:
A pencil (optional)

Directions:
If you would like to, use a sharp pencil to write what you would like to attract or manifest into your life onto the surface of the nasturtium and basil leaves. Or write something that you believe in and want to see more of in your life. You will be surprised how easy it is. Take as much time as you need to complete it, and enjoy every minute.

Combine the nuts, lemon juice, and garlic in a food processor and pulse until well chopped.

Add the nasturtium and basil leaves, and the cheese, and pulse again until combined.

Slowly add the olive oil while the food processor is running. This will help it to emulsify and keep the olive oil from separating.

Season to taste with salt and pepper, toss through your pasta, and enjoy!

CLOVES AND WINE
FOR GOOD LUCK

When my partner and I were looking for a house, nothing seemed to work. It felt as though our perfect house just did not exist, and that all the other witches had a bigger wallet than me. So I decided to call on Lady Luck by bathing in sweet aroma of clove. That night, in my dreams, I saw a perfect little house standing in a field of chamomile, and only three weeks later we bought the most perfect house with a huge chamomile bush by the front door. Not exactly a field, but it will do for now.

If you want to attract more luck and abundance into your life, try adding a few spoonfuls of cloves to your bathtub, burn cloves in your workplace, keep cloves in your pocket as an amulet, or try making this aromatic wine with cloves and other spices. Nowadays, cloves are also appreciated for their anti-inflammatory and antimicrobial properties, and are used in oral care and as a digestion aid.

Cloves have a rich history of use in luck, prosperity, and protection spells. There is a belief that these aromatic flower buds were so admired in Ancient Rome and China that they were prized more than gold!

Ingredients:
1 x 25 fl oz (750 ml) bottle of red wine (for a nonalcoholic version, use apple cider or apple juice)
6–8 whole cloves
2 oranges, sliced
¼ cup (60 ml) honey
2–3 cinnamon sticks
2–3 anise stars (optional)
1 tsp ground cardamom (optional)
¼ cup (60 ml) brandy (optional)

Directions:
Place all the ingredients in a saucepan over medium heat. As soon as the liquid begins to simmer, reduce the heat to low and cover.

Transform this mulled wine into a luck potion by giving it the occasional stir while whispering, "I deserve the best and it comes to me at the right time; I am grateful for all the opportunities in my life; I strengthen my good luck with good actions."

Let the elixir simmer (rather than boil) for 30 minutes.

Strain the mixture into glasses and serve immediately. You could use the leftover orange slices or cinnamon sticks to garnish.

As you sip this aromatic potion, envision yourself getting everything you wish for and imagine how good that feels.

VIOLET SUGAR FOR BLUE DAYS

Wild violets are the true heralds of spring—and the flowers and leaves of this simple but magnificent plant are completely edible and full of antioxidants.

Violet sugar is a magical way to capture the essence of spring—the excitement, the thrill, the enthusiasm, the love, the pleasure. You can use it in baking, add it to your tea, make a sugar rim for your cocktails, or add a few drops of your favorite oil to it to create a gentle sugar scrub for your beautiful skin. You can then use it throughout the year any time you need a pick-me-up, a dose of sunshine to brighten your day, or a little love on a blue day.

Foraging for your food is an almost spiritual experience. It provides an opportunity to slow down and really tune in with nature. But before you grab your basket, make sure you are aware of the unwritten rules of foraging: Know your local environment—you would be surprised how many plants are currently "at risk." Only harvest plants you can 100 percent identify. Do not harvest from roadsides or city parks. And never take more than you need. The rule of thumb is that you only harvest one-third of any particular patch, so plants can easily recover.

Ingredients:
1 cup (20 g) violet flowers, ideally freshly harvested, though store-bought fresh or dried organic flowers are also good
2 cups (400 g) white sugar

Equipment:
16 oz (450 ml) glass jar with lid
journal and pen (optional)

Directions:
Wash the flowers in cold water, then allow them to dry on some paper towel. Make sure the flowers are completely dry before moving on to the next step.

In a food processor, combine the flowers and sugar (the suggested ratio is one part flowers to two parts sugar).

Spread the mixture in a thin layer on a tray and allow to dry for several hours, stirring occasionally.

While the sugar is drying out, think of all the things that make you excited about the spring. What are you looking forward to? Say it out loud. Let your thoughts and words infuse the sugar with an aura of excitement and anticipation.

If desired, grab your journal and make a bucket list for the coming spring. And make sure to put self-love and self-care on that list.

Store the sugar in the jar, lid tightly closed, in a cool, dry place.

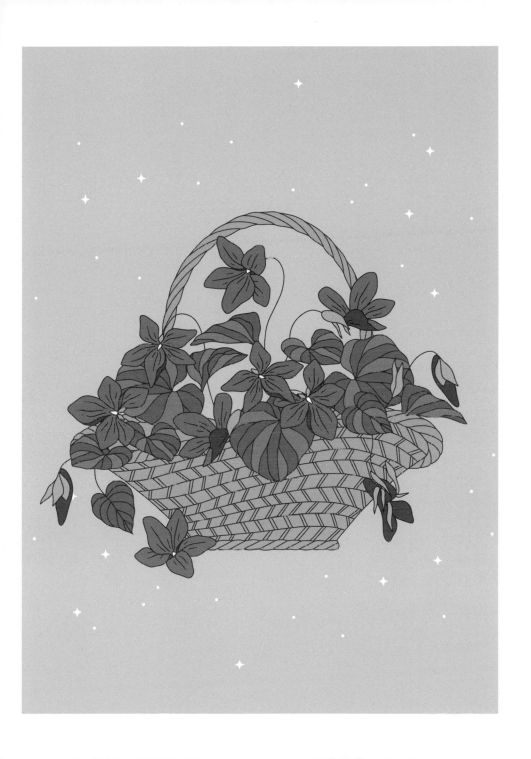

FIRE CIDER FOR HEX-BREAKING AND GOOD HEALTH

Fire cider is a cold-weather tonic made with herbs and apple cider vinegar. It has been around for decades, and naturally protects against colds and boosts your immune system.

One of my special ingredients is cayenne pepper, which is known to improve metabolism and fight infections. It is also a natural painkiller. In the witchy community, cayenne pepper is used in spells to repel negativity and unwanted energy and, of course, for hex-breaking!

Sometimes our inner dialogue of negative, judgmental self-talk is so loud that it makes us question our confidence and sense of self-worth. Try to remember that these thoughts and feelings may come and go, but our underlying sense of worth and love is always present within us. And if you ever need support in breaking negative thought patterns, and want to boost your confidence and immunity at the same time, try making this flavorful fire cider. As you take a spoonful of this potion, repeat the words: "I will only speak words of love to myself. I release all doubts and insecurities about myself."

Ingredients:
1 whole cayenne pepper
½ cup (50 g) fresh ginger, diced or shredded
¼ cup (25 g) fresh turmeric, diced or shredded, or 2 tbsp turmeric powder
½ cup (50 g) fresh horseradish, diced or shredded
6 garlic cloves, minced
1 lemon, cut into quarters
2 tbsp chopped fresh rosemary or 1 tsp dried
2 tbsp chopped fresh thyme or 1 tsp dried
1 tsp black peppercorns
3 cups (720 ml) apple cider vinegar
honey, to taste

Equipment:
2 x 32 oz (950 ml) glass jars with lids
cheesecloth (or other piece of fabric) and funnel, for straining

Directions:

Place all the ingredients except the cider vinegar and honey in a jar.

Fill the jar with the cider vinegar. It should cover the herbs by an inch or two.

Close the lid of the jar tightly. Use a piece of parchment paper under the lid to keep the vinegar from touching the metal, or use a plastic lid instead.

Let the mixture sit in a cool, dark place to infuse for at least 3–4 weeks. Shake once daily.

Strain the vinegar through cheesecloth into a clear jar. Do not rush it; let it drain for a good 15–20 minutes. And make sure to squeeze out every drop of this precious liquid.

Sweeten with honey to taste.

Store in a cool, dark place for up to a year. Shake well before using. Since fire cider is made with apple cider vinegar and honey, two of nature's great preservatives, it doesn't need to be refrigerated

Ways to enjoy fire cider:
- *Take 1–2 tbsp daily as an immune booster, especially during the cold and flu season.*
- *Add a spoonful to your water, tea, juice, or any other drink of your choice. It is very good with a Bloody Mary cocktail!*
- *Use it as a marinade or salad dressing.*
- *Try 1 tbsp as a hangover cure.*

SUNSHINE TINCTURE

The California poppy is the fastest-growing flower in my garden, and one of the first to awaken in spring—I like to think it's just so excited to share its gifts and medicine with us! This bright yellow flower truly embodies the energy of the sun, and is known for promoting restful sleep, easing anxiety and stress, and for calming and supporting the entire nervous system.

One of the easiest and safest potions you can make using California poppy is a tincture—a concentrated herbal extract. It can be taken straight by the dropper or diluted in tea or another beverage of your choice. I personally like to add tinctures to my homemade cocktails.

California poppy can be helpful for someone who wants to get out of their comfort zone—to shine their light, share their gifts, and be more open to the opportunities around them. This fearless little flower helps to awake that excitement and love of life.

Ingredients:
1 cup (40 g) fresh California poppy flowers and leaves or ½ cup (20 g) dried flowers
1 cup (240 ml) brandy (or any other 80-proof alcohol) or apple cider vinegar

Equipment:
8 oz (225 ml) glass jar
cheesecloth (or other piece of fabric) and funnel, for straining
dropper bottle, for storage (preferably a cobalt or amber glass bottle, to protect the liquid from sun exposure)

Directions:
Fill the jar three-quarters full with the fresh flowers. If you are working with dried flowers, fill the jar half full. (And if using apple cider vinegar in the next step, use dried flowers.)

Pour the alcohol or vinegar to the very top of the jar, covering the flowers completely.

Leave the mixture to extract for 6–8 weeks.

Strain the tincture through the cheesecloth into the dropper bottle.

Store in a cool, dark place and use within a year.

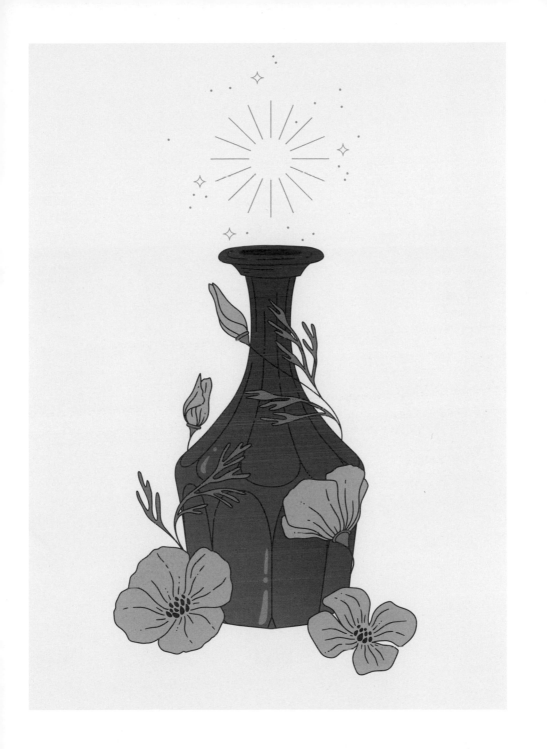

SHORTBREAD COOKIES FOR ENTHUSIASM AND ZEST FOR LIFE

Cornflowers, also known as "bachelor's buttons," are one of my favorite flowers to grow. The flowers and seeds can tolerate cold temperatures, they make fantastic cut flowers, and, if dried properly, they keep their beautiful vivid color.

Cornflowers are symbols of love, the passion of youth, and enthusiasm—an old tale says that they were once worn by men in love to show that they were single and had a romantic interest in a woman. Nowadays, herbalists use cornflowers to treat fever, water retention, and menstrual cramps. But in addition to their healing properties, they are the perfect flowers for all your kitchen potions—they are 100 percent edible, delicious, and their bright colors make spectacular garnishes for salads and drinks. And, of course, they are ideal for baking—so turn off your phone, put some good music on, admire the flowers, and savor every second of the cooking process.

Ingredients:
1 cup (225 g) unsalted butter
  (at room temperature)
½ tsp vanilla extract
½ cup (100 g) sugar
½ tsp kosher salt (optional)
½ tbsp grated orange zest
½ tbsp grated lemon zest
2 cups (240 g) all-purpose (plain) flour
1 large egg white, lightly beaten
handful of cornflowers, fresh or dried

Directions:
Beat together the butter and vanilla extract until creamed—you could do this by hand or in a food processor. Add the sugar, salt, and citrus zest and mix until combined.

Slowly add the flour, 1 cup (120 g) at a time, stopping occasionally to scrape down the sides of the bowl if using a processor.

Shape the dough—which should be moist but firm—into a rectangular block. Wrap it in plastic wrap (cling film) and chill in the refrigerator until firm enough to roll (about 1–2 hours is fine, although I like to chill it overnight).

Once the dough is ready, preheat the oven to 300°F (150°C). Baking at a fairly low temperature will help you preserve the color of the flowers. Roll out the dough to a maximum of ¼-inch (5 mm) thickness and use a cookie cutter to cut out shapes from the dough.

Place the cookies at least an inch (2.5 cm) apart on a baking sheet lined with parchment paper.

Using a pastry brush, gently brush a thin layer of beaten egg white onto the center of each cookie. Then gently press a flower blossom (or just a few petals) onto the surface. (Alternatively, press the flowers onto the cookies straight after baking—the heat will help the petals stick.)

Place the sheet into the fridge for 10–15 minutes, to make sure the dough is cold, before transferring to the oven and baking for 10–15 minutes until lightly golden and smelling delicious!

Allow the cookies to cool—and enjoy.

There is much evidence of the use of cornflowers throughout history in different parts of the world. In England, monks made cornflower wine to treat flu, coughs, and kidney diseases. In France, they were commonly used as a compress to relieve eye strain. And it is also believed that these blue flowers were used in Ancient Egypt to decorate the altars of pharaohs.

BASIL SALT FOR PROSPERITY AND LOVE

Basil is known as the "king of herbs," with antibacterial, anti-inflammatory, and healing properties. It is incredibly good for the digestive and nervous systems, and a simple basil tea is a great remedy for a headache.

Basil has strong ties to abundance, good fortune, money, love, and protection. The first written mention of basil dates back to the third century BCE, and there are numerous stories and legends connected with this magical herb—some declaring it a poison, others a cure. But the two main spiritual properties of basil have remained the same: prosperity and love. Even today, basil is one of the favorite witchy herbs for abundance spells. Place a dried or pressed piece of basil in your wallet and watch your money grow. Or run a hot bath and add a handful of basil leaves to increase your magnetism. And try making this magical basil salt—you can use it to enhance the flavors of a dish, and to attract more prosperity and love into your everyday life.

Ingredients:
½ cup (12 g) fresh or dried basil
1 cup (280 g) coarse sea salt
a few rose petals, for extra magic (optional)

Equipment:
8 oz (225 ml) glass jar with lid

Directions:
Wash the basil in cold water and dry it well. If using fresh basil, chop the leaves and stems into small pieces.

Put the salt and basil into a blender and blitz for a minute, or until completely smooth.

Spread the mixture evenly on a baking sheet, and place in the oven for 15–20 minutes at the lowest temperature that your oven allows (around 200–250°F/95–120°C), stirring once or twice during baking.

Store the salt in the glass jar with the lid tightly shut. For best flavor, use within three months.

In Romanian folklore, if a young man accepts a sprig of basil from a young woman, he will fall madly in love with her. The Greeks and Romans believed the most potent basil could only be grown if the seed was sowed while cursing.

GINGER OXYMEL FOR INCREASING PERSONAL POWER

Ginger is truly one of the most potent plants out there. Many love and abundance spells contain ginger, and we all know of its healing abilities—it has anti-inflammatory and antiviral properties, and is one of the best plants to aid with digestion. There are many potions you can make using ginger, from a simple tea to syrup, or even a tincture, but my favorite, especially during the winter months, is an oxymel.

An oxymel is a herbal remedy that has been around for centuries, and is a simple mixture of honey, vinegar, and medicinal herbs. It takes a few weeks to make, but I promise you it is worth it. Use it to ignite your inner fire, to calm an upset stomach, and to support a healthy immune system. Take 1–2 teaspoons daily, and repeat the words: "I am healthy and strong, filled with passion and drive, I have the power to create joy, abundance, and success in my life." You could also come up with your own affirmations.

Ingredients:
2-inch (5 cm) piece fresh ginger root, sliced into strips or rounds
1 cup (240 ml) apple cider vinegar
1 cup (240 ml) honey

Equipment:
2 x 16 oz (450 ml) glass jars with lids
fine-mesh strainer

Directions:
Fill a jar one-third full with the ginger.

Fill the jar about half full with apple cider vinegar and the remaining half with honey. Fill the jar as full as you can without it overflowing. Too much airspace at the top will cause oxidation and make the ginger turn brown.

Fasten the lid of the jar and give it a good shake, then let it infuse for 1–4 weeks. If you are using a metal lid, be sure to put a piece of parchment paper underneath it, to prevent the vinegar reacting with the metal.

Using a fine-mesh strainer, strain the oxymel into a clean jar for storage, discarding the ginger. Store the oxymel in a cool place out of direct sunlight and use within six months.

Ginger is associated with the energy of the sun and inner fire. In magical spells it is used as a catalyst, to speed up the desired outcome. It is also used to increase a person's inner energy and magical powers.

CACAO AND BLUE LOTUS TO AWAKEN THE THIRD EYE

Blue lotus grows in water and is often confused with water lilies. Its bright purple flowers were sacred to Ancient Egyptians—they were believed to have anti-aging properties and were used in cosmetics. More importantly, blue lotus was used in ceremonies to enter higher states of consciousness or deepen the meditative state. This mystical flower has the dual effect of awakening and relaxing—both at the same time.

Nowadays, modern witches use blue lotus as a sleep aid, anxiety reliever, aphrodisiac, and lucid dreaming enhancer. It is also a third eye opener. Here, the soothing and sweet cacao complements the earthy and bitter taste of blue lotus and makes the perfect restorative drink for any time of the day or night.

The third eye is your invisible eye, located between the eyebrows. It is a representation of your intuition and inner wisdom, allowing you to see things as they truly are, beyond ordinary sight. So, if you ever find yourself at a crossroads, struggling to make a decision, or desperately looking for the right direction and answer, try blue lotus. Not only will it help you to see things from a different perspective, but it will awaken your intuition and provide you with an opportunity to listen to your soul.

Ingredients:
1 tsp dried blue lotus flowers
¼ cup (60 ml) just-boiled water
1½ tbsp raw cacao powder
¼–½ cup (60–120 ml) warm milk of your choice
1 tbsp coconut cream (optional)
1 tsp sugar (optional)

Equipment:
fine-mesh strainer
journal and pen

Directions:
Steep the blue lotus flowers in the just-boiled water for 3–5 minutes. Blue lotus has a very potent taste, so try not to overdo the suggested amount since it can make your elixir taste bitter.

While the blue lotus tea is brewing, add the remaining ingredients to your favorite mug and whisk thoroughly.

Strain the tea and add it to the mug.

Find a comfortable seat and, on a completely blank page of your journal, write down a problem that you can't seem to find a solution for, or a question that has been keeping you awake at night.

As you sip the potion, observe your thoughts, and see if anything changes. Your hand may pick up the pen and start channeling your inner wisdom, shining a light on all the answers that have been within you the whole time.

LIQUID COURAGE

For thousands of years, thyme was a symbol of courage and bravery in many European societies. The Ancient Greeks, for example, added thyme to their bath water and used it in incense at their places of worship. Today, thyme is used to address many respiratory and digestive issues—and in the kitchen, it can enhance the flavors of any dish. Thyme essential oil is believed to help with concentration.

If you ever find yourself feeling stuck or afraid, anxious to move on or start doing something new, try this lunar thyme infusion for an instant boost of courage.

During the Middle Ages, women would give thyme leaves as gifts to knights departing for war, because it was believed to fight off melancholy and bring great courage to the wearer.

Ingredients:
a few sprigs of fresh thyme
water, as needed

Equipment:
2 x 8 oz (225 ml) glass jars with lids
cheesecloth (or other piece of fabric)
  and funnel, for straining

Directions:
Place the thyme sprigs into a glass jar, then fill the jar with water while repeating the words: "I am choosing courage over comfort, I am choosing confidence over doubt, I am choosing me." Seal the jar tightly.

Place the jar outside in the moonlight overnight to allow the thyme to infuse its properties into the water.

In the morning, strain the liquid into a clean jar and store in the fridge until ready to use (make sure to use it within a few days). You can drink this liquid courage, add it to your bath water, or use it as a hair rinse.

MOON MILK FOR DEEP REST

Moon milk, as the name implies, is a potion to be enjoyed just before going to bed. Also known as golden milk, it is a well-known Ayurvedic drink made with milk and spices, encouraging deep rest any time your emotions are running high, when you feel the energy around you amplified, or when your immune system needs a boost. There are literally dozens of variations of this fantastic potion, with some containing over 15 different spices.

The three main components are milk, turmeric, and my secret ingredient: ashwagandha. Ashwagandha is famous for its anti-inflammatory and antistress properties and has been known to help lower cortisol levels and anxiety. So, allow yourself to slow down, postpone your to-do list and have some quality rest with a cup of hot moon milk.

Ashwagandha is native to India and Nepal, but can be grown in your backyard in average soil. I have been growing this medicinal root for the last five years and it is such a magical experience. It takes around two years for the root to become fully grown and ready to harvest. It doesn't rush, taking deep, long rests during its growth, sometimes sleeping for months. But it goes through every phase with grace.

Ingredients:
2 cups (480 ml) milk of your choice
½ tsp ground ashwagandha powder
½ tsp ground turmeric
⅛ tsp ground ginger
⅛ tsp ground cinnamon
pinch of ground nutmeg
pinch of black pepper
1 tsp coconut oil or ghee
1 tsp honey or another sweetener (optional)
a few dried rose petals (optional)

Directions:
Pour the milk into a medium saucepan and bring it to a low simmer. Do not allow it to boil.

Once the milk is hot, add the rest of the ingredients, except the oil or ghee and the honey or sweetener. Give it a good stir and simmer gently for 5 minutes. As you simmer this aromatic potion, think of the aspects of your life that are calling you to soften, to surrender more, to love more.

Lastly, stir through the coconut oil or ghee, add honey or other sweetener, if desired, sprinkle over some rose petals, and serve immediately.

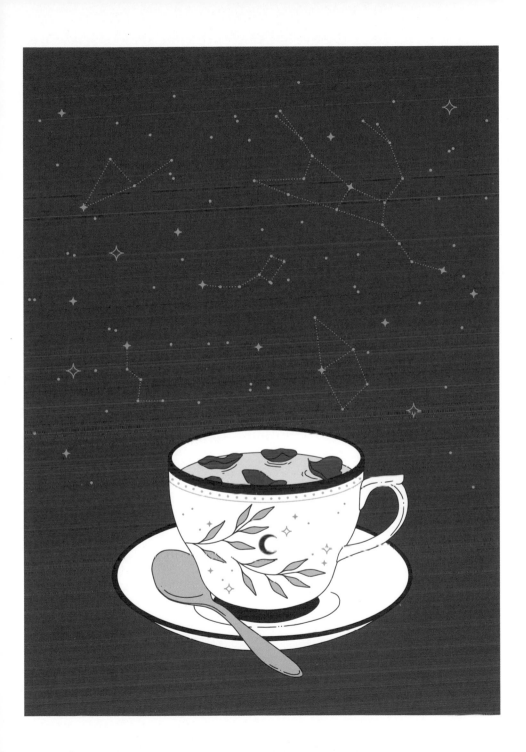

COMFORTING
MARSHMALLOW INFUSION

In the witchy world, marshmallow is known as the plant that turns things into gold (quite literally sometimes, since the root turns water a light yellow color). It is deeply connected with love, fertility, and rebirth, since it is believed that marshmallow holds feminine energy, and there are stories of people planting marshmallow seeds under the light of the full moon in an attempt to get pregnant.

Today, marshmallow is known as a calming and soothing plant, used to help with heartburn, stomach ache, and a sore throat, and is widely used in cosmetics and skincare. Witches call it a comforting plant, because its viscous texture literally hugs you from the inside. And this cold-water infusion is a perfect example of that. Make it any time you feel down, lonely, or under the weather. And as you sip it, envision a bright yellow light enveloping you, hugging you outside and in, giving love and light to every cell in your body.

Ingredients:
½ cup marshmallow root or ¼ cup
  marshmallow root powder

Equipment:
2 x 16 oz (450 ml) glass jars with lid
cheesecloth (or other piece of fabric)
  and funnel, for straining

Directions:
Fill a jar a quarter full with marshmallow root.

Add cold water until the jar is full, close the lid, and leave to infuse overnight. The marshmallow will do its magic and turn the water into a thick and viscous elixir.

In the morning, strain the liquid into a clean jar, discarding the roots.

Add the infusion to your tea or water, or take a few droplets straight up. You can also use it to rinse your hair—marshmallow infusion is nature's best conditioner and is incredibly good for dry or brittle hair.

Store in the fridge and use within three days.

The first marshmallows were prepared by boiling roots of the marshmallow plant with honey (before gelatin took over). Marshmallow root contains natural mucilage, which gives marshmallows the fluffy texture we all love. It is believed that the Ancient Egyptians were the first to notice the incredible properties of this plant, using it for respiratory problems and to treat a sore throat, cough, asthma, and bronchitis.

LEMON BALM SPRITZER
TO HEAL A BROKEN HEART

This is one of the most popular potions around. You'd think, then, that by now there would be the perfect recipe for it, with just the right ingredients, but unfortunately not. Every witch knows that there is no herb and no potion strong enough to offer an instant cure for a broken heart. But there are some herbs that can soothe your pain, help with insomnia, and lighten your weight, and one of them is calming lemon balm. No matter how big or small a heartbreak you are going through, give yourself time to grieve and heal. Try not to numb the feelings, but experience all the emotions. Ask for help if needed. And just let it all go.

Lemon balm is known to reduce stress and anxiety, promote restful sleep, even improve appetite and ease stomach pain. Sometimes when I feel down, I go to my garden and just sit there and smell the lemon balm. The earthy, minty aroma always helps to ground me and clear the brain fog.

Ingredients:
1 cup (150 g) fresh or frozen blackberries
½ cup (120 ml) honey (or use maple or agave syrup)
¼ cup (60 ml) freshly squeezed lemon juice
1 cup (25 g) fresh lemon balm leaves, plus extra for garnish
2 lemons, cut into wedges
sparkling water
ice, to serve

Equipment:
cheesecloth (or other piece of fabric) or a fine-mesh strainer, for straining

Directions:
Place the blackberries, honey, and lemon juice in a medium saucepan. Cook over low heat for about 5 minutes, or until the blackberries become mushy. Strain the mixture through cheesecloth or a fine-mesh strainer into a bowl, using the back of a spoon to squeeze the juice from the blackberries. Allow the juice to cool, then chill in the refrigerator.

Using a muddler (a type of pestle) or spoon, mash the lemon balm with the lemon wedges, then refrigerate until chilled.

Once chilled, combine the blackberry mixture and lemon mixture in a pitcher, and fill with cold sparkling water.

Serve over ice, garnished with lemon balm leaves.

COSMOS PUNCH FOR HARMONY

Cosmos is one of the easiest edible flowers to grow, and has many medicinal uses. It is believed to boost the immune system and help with skin conditions. In Brazil, cosmos flowers have even been used to treat malaria.

They are also the perfect flowers to gift to your loved ones, whether friends, family, or romantic partners. No special occasion is required—they just symbolize harmony and the idea of walking hand in hand together through life, experiencing all of the joys it brings. So let the drinking of this punch create the deep, harmonious, and meaningful connections that we all so desperately need.

The name "cosmos" was given by Spanish priests who originally grew the flowers during their missions abroad. They were amazed by the petals, which were all the same size and placed so evenly. As a result, they named the flowers "cosmos" to symbolize their order, balance, and harmony with the rest of the Universe.

Ingredients:
2 lb (900 g) fresh berries (blackberries, strawberries, raspberries, etc.)
1½ cups (360 ml) water
1 cup (240 ml) honey or 1½ cups (300 g) sugar
juice of 10–12 lemons (around 1–1½ cups/ 240–360 ml)
1 tsp rosewater (optional)
4 cups (960 ml) sparkling water
handful of cosmos flowers
ice, to serve
lemon balm or mint leaves, for garnish (optional)

Directions:
In a blender, purée the berries to a smooth consistency (you might need to add a little water). Set aside.

In a small saucepan over medium heat, combine the 1½ cups (360 ml) water with the honey or sugar and simmer until it dissolves. Do not allow the water to boil.

Combine the lemon juice, berry purée, honey syrup, and rosewater, if using, in a jug. Give this a good stir and set aside in the refrigerator for an hour or so.

Pour the chilled lemonade mixture into a punch bowl and add the sparkling water.

Add the cosmos flowers. With every flower you add, think of the people you are going to share this punch with, and speak words of love and harmony. Send a blessing their way. Or tell the flowers the joys of life you want to experience and what you are looking forward to.

Serve over ice, garnished with lemon balm or mint leaves, if desired.

CRISPY SAGE LEAVES FOR CLARITY

Every path, every goal, and every mission starts with clarity and a clear vision. After all, if you don't know what you want, it is impossible to obtain or request it. Simple garden sage has been known to promote mental clarity, remove brain fog, and improve mood. It is also famous for its antiseptic properties, making it one of the best remedies for a sore throat.

One of the easiest ways to enjoy sage is by making a tea or a simple cold-water infusion. But if you want to try something different, make these crispy sage leaves. Add them to your favorite dishes or pop one in your mouth for an instant dose of clarity and wisdom. Pure magic.

No matter where you are on your journey, if you need a vision for next month or even next year, try the medicine of this ancient plant. The very word "sage" means a wise man. So, in many folklore stories, it is associated with wisdom and immortality.

Ingredients:
¼ cup (60 ml) olive oil
handful of fresh sage leaves
coarse sea salt, for sprinkling

Directions:
Heat the oil in a frying pan over medium-high heat. It is very important to get the oil hot before adding the sage. If the sage doesn't sizzle when you add it to the oil, it is not hot enough.

Fry the sage leaves for 1 minute, then flip them over and fry for an additional 30 seconds to 1 minute until crispy.

Remove the leaves from the pan and lay them on paper towel to soak up the excess oil.

Sprinkle generously with salt and serve immediately, or keep in the fridge for up to three days. Use them to garnish your pasta or meat; crush and add them to soups or salad dressings; and my favorite thing is to add them to homemade gnocchi along with walnuts.

FORGET-ME-NOT SALAD

Compared to other flowers, forget-me-nots don't hold that many medicinal properties. So the question as to why these humble flowers occupied so many minds in the past remains unanswered to this day. Forget-me-nots represent true love, devotion, and being true to yourself. They make a great gift for someone when you want them to keep you in mind. And their magical power is to help you remember (or to not-forget) your intentions, desires, and all the important things we tend to forget when life gets busy. In addition to all its witchy properties, forget-me-nots are completely edible and make a great addition to most kitchen spells.

There are dozens of legends about these tiny, bright, mysterious blooms, some of them dating back thousands of years. One of the most famous is an old German story about how these beautiful flowers got their name. It tells of how God was naming all the plants one afternoon, and one tiny but courageous plant that was still unnamed called out to God, saying: "Forget me not, O Lord!" In response, God named the plant with the very same words.

Ingredients:
your favorite salad ingredients
dash of your favorite salad dressing
handful of fresh forget-me-not flowers

Equipment:
journal and pen (optional)

Directions:
Start by making your favorite salad. Not your partner's favorite, not your kids' favorite. Make the most perfect salad for YOURSELF.

Add a dash of your favorite dressing and sprinkle over the forget-me-nots. As you sprinkle these beautiful tiny flowers, say out loud all the things that you keep forgetting sometimes, whatever it might be: Forget-me-not to be patient with myself; Forget-me-not to love myself every second of the day; Forget-me-not that my journey doesn't have to look a certain way; Forget-me-not to always make time for myself; Forget-me-not that I always deserve the best; Forget-me-not to treat myself...

Write all of these things down in your journal, if desired. When we write things down, we are more likely to remember them and take action.

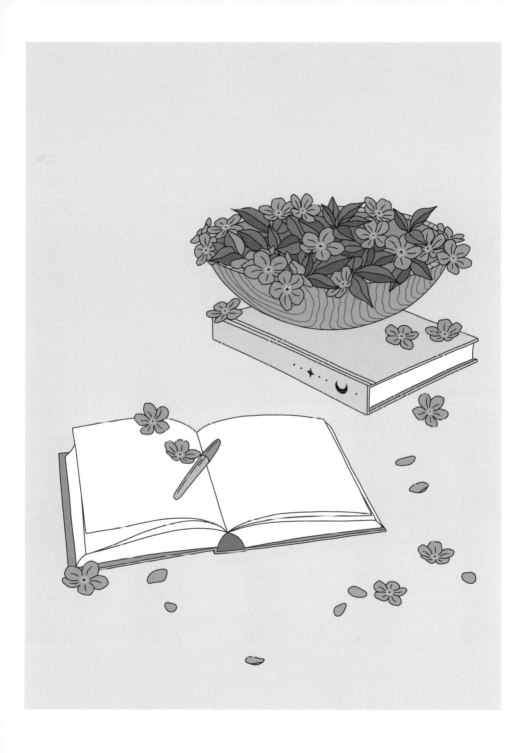

MAGICAL ICED TEA
FOR PSYCHIC ABILITIES

We all have psychic abilities, a sixth sense, intuition, and the power to heal; some people just choose to trust their inner knowledge more, and some of us need help and guidance in that area. Fear and self-doubt are the biggest elements that prevent us from exploring our abilities—fear of judgment from others, and the inability to fully trust ourselves. So if you want to tap into the unknown, try to let go of fear and choose the brave path. And to enhance your psychic abilities, try this magical blue butterfly pea tea.

Blue butterfly pea flower is special for many reasons—it is known as a brain herb and has been used for centuries to enhance memory and treat anxiety and depression. It is high in antioxidants, and is also used to aid digestion and treat respiratory problems. But what makes this fascinating plant stand out are its transformational properties. When you add the flowers to water, they immediately release their beautiful blue color. And if you add an acid, such as lemon juice, the color will change again—from blue to gorgeous magenta. So ask yourself—what can you add to your life to bring more color, excitement, magic, and love? How can you allow yourself to change mood, job, interests—anything—without judgment from yourself?

Ingredients:
1–2 tbsp butterfly pea flowers
1 cup (240 ml) just-boiled water
1 cup ice
dash of honey (optional)
lemon slice

Equipment:
journal and pen (optional)

Directions:

Add the flowers to the cup of just-boiled water.

Leave the tea to brew for 5–10 minutes, then strain and discard the flowers. The longer you steep the flowers in hot water, the deeper and brighter the color will be. Use the back of a spoon to press the flowers against the cup to extract more color, if desired.

Pour the tea over the ice and add sweeteners of your choice, such as honey.

Add the lemon slice and watch the magic happen.

As you sip your tea, reflect on the questions you asked yourself. Perhaps you might choose to record your thoughts in a journal.

Psychic abilities can present themselves in many different forms. Have you ever turned around because you felt someone staring at you? Or thought of something or someone, and the next thing you know you run into that person or found that thing on the side of the road? These are examples of an intuitive psychic gift in action.

ELDERFLOWER POPSICLES FOR EMOTIONAL HEALING

The elder tree is known as a "whole medicine chest" and has been used by herbalists and witches to help with physical and emotional healing. The aroma of elderflowers is probably one of my favorite smells in the whole word, soothing the heart, filling it with love, and helping you heal any spiritual and emotional issues. No wonder these magnificent flowers are used in spells for hex-breaking.

One of the easiest ways to attract the magical and healing properties of elderflower is by making a simple tea, but if you want to take your kitchen spells to the next level, try making these floral popsicles. They're great on a sizzling summer day, and the perfect way to support your healing journey and to add more love and joy to your day. You could use elderflower cordial instead of tea, if desired, for a more potent floral taste.

The incredible properties of elderberry syrup are well known, but did you know that all parts of the tree—its leaves, root, bark, and flowers—can be used for a whole range of purposes? For example, in folk herbalism the bark of young elder trees was used as a laxative and diuretic, while the leaves were cooked and transformed into a salve to treat bruises and inflammation.

Ingredients:
elderflower tea, enough for around 4 cups (960 ml) (standard 10–12 popsicle molds usually hold around 3 fl oz/90 ml each), or elderflower cordial
sugar, to taste
pinch of salt
1 tbsp freshly squeezed lemon juice or grated lemon zest (optional)
handful of fresh elderflowers and pansy petals (optional)

Equipment:
popsicle mold

Directions:
Start by making freshly brewed elderflower tea. Add sugar to your taste, a pinch of salt, and the lemon juice or zest, if desired, and let it brew for at least 15–20 minutes. If you are working with elderflower cordial, simply mix the cordial with water (the suggested ratio is 1:1).

Allow the mixture to cool, then pour into the molds. Make sure to leave some space at the top of the molds for the popsicles to expand. If desired, add a few fresh elderflower and pansy petals (or any other edible flowers of your choice) for an extra dose of magic and love.

Insert the popsicle sticks and freeze for at least four hours (or until completely hard).

If you have trouble removing your popsicles from the mold, simply run the mold under warm water for just a few seconds. Then enjoy these magical popsicles and let all your worries melt away!

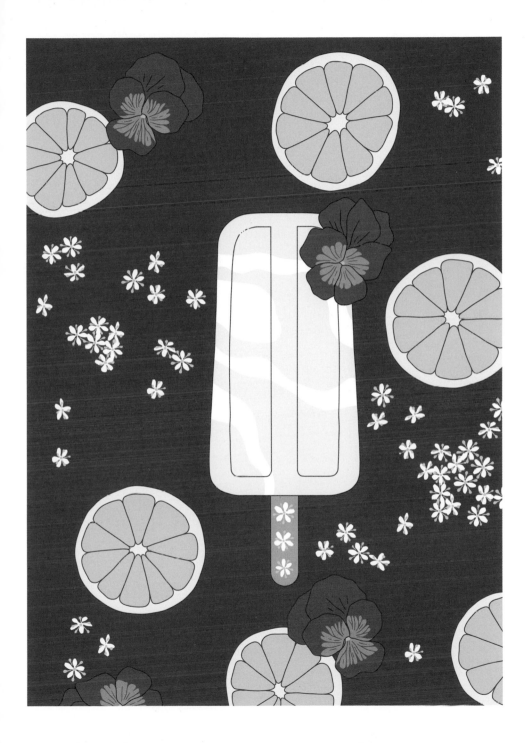

FLORAL CHOCOLATE BARK

What better way to treat yourself than with chocolate and flowers, and this simple recipe features both. Pansies symbolize love in all her forms—platonic, romantic, friendship, unconditional, and, of course, self-love.

In Shakespeare's famous comedy Midsummer Night's Dream, the juice of a pansy was used to make a love potion. This humble but bright and colorful flower offers so much vitality and everyday magic. They are very easy to grow, but the best part is that, even if you don't have a garden, pansies are the most common edible flowers—this means you will likely find them at your local urban farms. Some grocery stores even carry them during the summer season (remember only to purchase edible flowers from the produce section in the store, not the floral section).

Ingredients:
2 cups (340 g) chocolate chips of your choice (dark, milk, white, or a mix)
handful of dried pansy flowers
handful of your favorite dried berries, seeds, or nuts (optional)

Directions:
Start by melting the chocolate. You can either do this in a microwave, heating the chocolate in 30-second bursts, and stirring each time so as not to burn the chocolate; or on the stove, placing the chocolate in a heatproof bowl over a pan of simmering water—making sure the bowl is not touching the water—until the chocolate is melted.

Line a baking sheet with parchment paper and pour the melted chocolate onto it. Using a spatula or spoon, spread the chocolate into an even layer about ¼-inch (5 mm) thick.

Top your chocolate with the dried pansies. Add some dried berries, seeds, nuts, or any other toppings, if desired. Make sure to press them into the chocolate slightly.

Chill in the refrigerator for at least 30 minutes, or until the chocolate is completely hard. Use the back of your spatula or spoon to break the chocolate into pieces of bark, and enjoy!

ICE CUBES WITH ZINNIAS FOR JOYFUL ENDURANCE

Every gardener loves zinnias, since they are one of the easiest blooms to grow! They thrive in the summer heat and are unafraid of drought or bugs. This is why herbalists associate zinnias with determination, stoicism, and "joyful endurance." Joyful endurance is not about powering through difficult times, pushing yourself beyond your limits, postponing dreams, or neglecting other spheres of your life, but rather enjoying and loving life as it comes, with all its ups and downs, challenges, and surprises.

If you would like to preserve these little drops of joy for the months ahead, try making ice cubes with them. Zinnias keep their color well and will brighten up any drink with their presence!

Zinnias are completely edible and have an earthy and slightly sour taste. Sprinkle some petals in your salad or use them to garnish your favorite dish.

Ingredients:
handful of fresh zinnia petals (if you don't have any fresh zinnias handy, try other edible flowers instead)

Equipment:
ice cube tray

Directions:
Start by boiling water and then cooling it to room temperature once or twice. The boiling drives off dissolved gases, which makes the ice appear clearer.

Pour the warm water into the ice cube tray, filling each hole only half full.

Add zinnia petals to each hole of the ice cube tray and freeze overnight.

The following day, add more cooled boiled water, filling the holes to the top. This technique ensures that your beautiful flowers stay in the middle of the ice cube rather than on the surface. Freeze overnight again.

Any time you use these colorful floral ice cubes, remind yourself that life doesn't have to look a certain way. Every little bump is an important part of the journey. Allow yourself to grow and bloom in your own time.

CHIVE BLOSSOM BUTTER
FOR GOOD TIMES

Chives are associated with balance and harmony. Even their appearance is all about balance, harmony, and the union of opposites—because, let's be honest, what could be more bizarre than a green onion with delicious pink flowers? Mother Nature really does have her unique ways.

This tasty chive blossom butter is perfect for good times with friends or to savor on a relaxing solo evening. It will brighten up any simple bread basket or cheese platter and serve as a reminder of how two opposites can complement each other so well. And while you make this delicious treat, think about your own unique qualities, especially those that may appear contradictory or incompatible at first glance, but which, in reality, harmonize so well.

Ingredients:
1 cup (225 g) butter, softened
handful of chives, chopped
handful of chive blossoms, chopped

Directions:
In a bowl, combine the butter and half of your chives and chive blossoms. Mix thoroughly.

Next, lay a piece of plastic wrap (cling film) on your work surface. Mold your butter into a log and place it on top of the plastic wrap. Sprinkle the rest of the chives and blossoms over the butter, pressing them down gently and rolling the log in them to cover it completely.

Wrap the log in the plastic wrap, store in the fridge, and enjoy!

It is believed that in the Middle Ages, chives were used to lift the spirits of those who were feeling depressed, to protect from evil temptations, and to bring a sense of purpose. Witches used them in spells to help break negative habits and bring inner peace.

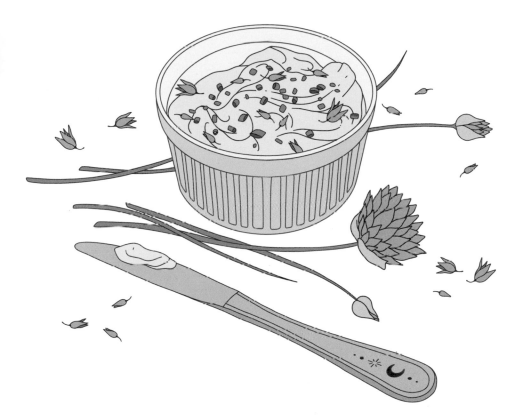

ROSE SYRUP FOR DEVOTION

The rose is known as the queen of the flower kingdom and is associated with love, passion, wisdom, beauty, and devotion. For thousands of years, cultures around the world have worshipped these beautiful and delicate flowers. They are a treat for our senses and eyes and give us much-needed medicine for the wounded heart. Roses are believed to be a great ally in helping to relieve anxiety, depression, and grief, and to bring a zest for life.

Any time you want to bring a little more sweetness and love into your life, try adding rose petals to your bath or using rose essential oil. Or if you would like to truly capture the essence of the rose, make this simple syrup, and whenever you feel down, just pour a few drops into your water, cocktail, or tea. Let the delicious taste and aroma inspire you and remind you to be loyal to yourself and—first and foremost—to love yourself.

In Greek mythology, the rose is associated with Aphrodite, goddess of love, and symbolizes love and beauty that will never fade—even through time or death.

Ingredients:
1 cup (240 ml) water
1 cup (200 g) white sugar
½ cup (20 g) fresh or dried rose petals
1 tbsp lemon juice
a few drops of pink food coloring (optional)

Equipment:
fine-mesh strainer
16 oz (450 ml) jar with lid

Directions:
Combine the water and sugar in a saucepan over medium heat, and heat until the sugar has dissolved completely.

Add the rose petals to the pan, reduce the heat and simmer for 10–15 minutes.

Add the lemon juice, turn off the heat, and leave to cool. The lemon juice will help to preserve the syrup and prevent it from crystallizing.

Strain the syrup through a fine-mesh strainer into the jar and discard the rose petals. Add a little food coloring, if desired, to enhance the color of the syrup.

Store in the fridge and use within a few weeks.

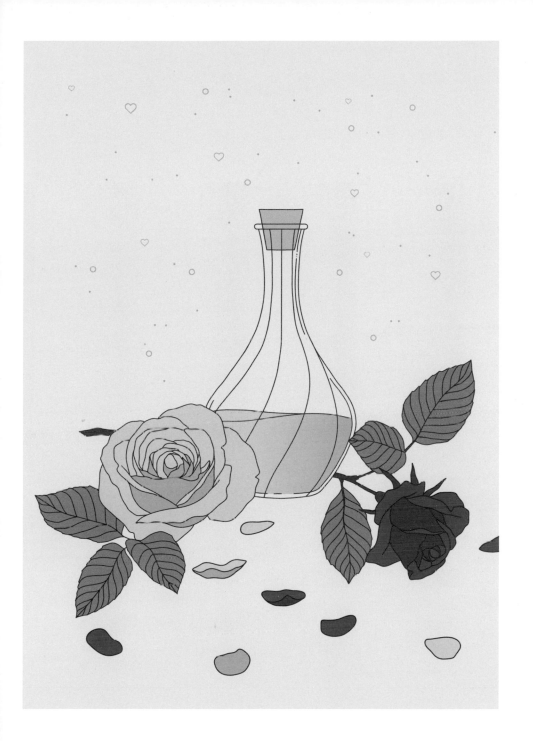

SUNFLOWER ELIXIR TO BRING BACK GOOD MEMORIES

I call this easy-to-make elixir "summer in a bottle." As with all other seasonal witchy medicine, it captures the essence, energy, mood, and potential of that season and allows you to savor it throughout the year. Summer is all about having fun—days are longer and more eventful, and there is an aura of excitement and endless possibility in the air.

Nothing symbolizes summer quite like sunflowers. They represent sun, warmth, and joy, but also self-confidence, to go for your wildest dreams. Day after day they follow the sun, from east to west, reminding us to trust our intuition, be loyal to ourselves, and follow our heart. Sunflower petals are also used in herbal teas and are believed to help with digestion, wound care, and even childbirth.

Ingredients:
handful of sunflower petals
2 cups (480 ml) distilled water
1 cup (240 ml) brandy (or any other 80-proof alcohol) or apple cider vinegar
dash of honey or another sweetener (optional)

Equipment:
16 oz (450 ml) glass jar with lid
journal and pen

Directions:

Wash and dry the fresh flower petals and place them in the jar.

Fill the jar with distilled water and close the lid tightly.

Let the elixir sit outside in the sun for a day (this is called solar infusion. If you feel more connected to the energy of the moon, leave the elixir out at night for lunar infusion).

Strain the elixir, discarding the flowers, and divide the elixir into two. One part is for you to drink that day, to invigorate your soul and charge every cell of your body with summer energy. The other is to preserve for later use.

To preserve the summer elixir, add the brandy or vinegar to the remaining elixir (the suggested ratio is 1:1). Feel free to add some honey or other sweetener to it. If using brandy, store in a dark, dry place. If using vinegar, store in the refrigerator. Drink a little or add a few drops to your water throughout the coming year to bring happy summer memories.

To complete this ritual, grab your journal and pen and write down your best summer memories—how wonderful the sunshine feels on your skin, how the long days of sunlight inspire you, and so on. Savor every word as you write and, as the days become colder and less eventful, enjoy a few drops of the sunflower elixir and come back to these pages. Read a paragraph or two and reignite your soul with the warm memories.

You can make this elixir with any edible summer blooming plant. Lavender, rosemary, mint, roses, calendula, chamomile, lemon balm, sage blossom, sweet peas, marigolds, zinnias—all are great options bursting with the summer energy of joy and happiness.

HONEY-FERMENTED GARLIC
TO WARD OFF EVIL SPIRITS

It's no surprise that witches have always loved garlic! It wasn't just used to repel vampires and evil spirits, but also envy and jealousy. Witches would bless their new homes by hanging some garlic. Brides would carry cloves of garlic in their pockets to bring them luck. Sailors would take garlic on long voyages to protect against wreckage and drowning. But most importantly, garlic was known (and still is) for its powerful healing properties in treating colds and flu, lowering blood pressure, fighting bacteria, treating ear infections, helping with certain skin conditions, and much more.

If, like me, you want the benefits of garlic but can't tolerate the pungent taste, try making honey-fermented garlic, one of the easiest fermentation recipes there is.

Ingredients:
1 cup (240 ml) honey
2 heads of garlic, cloves peeled
   and crushed or cut in half

Equipment:
16 oz (450 ml) glass jar with airtight glass or
   plastic lid

Directions:

Add the honey and garlic to the jar.

Seal the jar with the lid and turn it upside down (feel free to place a plate beneath the jar, just in case!).

Within a few days, you will see air bubbles forming and the honey becoming watery. This is a sign of active fermentation. For the next two weeks, open the jar daily to release excess carbon dioxide. Just a quick opening of the lid is more than enough to release the gases (some call it "burping the jar"). If for some reason the fermentation doesn't begin, add 1-2 tsp water to the mixture to help with the process.

After two weeks, the fermented garlic is ready to enjoy. For an even smoother taste, I recommend fermenting garlic for 4–5 weeks.

Store your fermented garlic in the fridge and use within six months.

There are many ways to enjoy this fermented garlic and honey:
- Any time you find yourself feeling envious or jealous, pop a clove of garlic into your mouth. Let it banish all the negative vibes and remind you that envy is just the recognition that you want something. So feel it all. Do not be hard on yourself. Recognize your desires. And start taking action.
- Use the garlic and honey to top your hummus or any other dip.
- Use the honey in salad dressings and marinades.
- Any time you have a sore throat (or as a preventative), eat one of the garlic cloves or a spoonful of the infused honey. The fermentation will sweeten and mellow the garlic taste, making it a delicious treat.

SPRING MAGNOLIA COCKTAIL FOR ETERNAL LOVE

The beauty and fragrance of magnolia can only be associated with spring. Magnolia might look delicate and fragile, but in reality it is a very tough and resilient flower. So it's no surprise that magnolia flowers represent endurance, life force, and eternal love. If you are ever able to get your hands on magnolia blossoms, treat yourself to a wonderful cocktail, and with every sip welcome more love and light into your heart, and celebrate the return of spring.

According to recent archeological excavations in America, in order to survive, magnolia trees have been adapting to Earth's changing climactic and geological conditions for millions of years. Yes, millions!

Ingredients:
handful of magnolia petals
ice
1 fl oz (30 ml) tequila (for a nonalcoholic version, use your favorite juice and sparkling water in place of the tequila and wine)
½ cup (120 ml) rose wine
1 fl oz (30 ml) freshly squeezed lime juice, plus 1 wedge of lime
½ –1 oz (15–30 g) simple syrup (depending on how sweet you like your cocktails)
pink Himalayan salt for the rim (optional)

Equipment:
cocktail shaker or mason jar with lid

Directions:
Wash your magnolia petals in cold water, then leave them to dry on a paper towel.

Fill the cocktail shaker (or jar) with ice, add the tequila, wine, lime juice, and simple syrup, and shake vigorously.

Rub the lime wedge around the rim of a glass and dip the rim into the Himalayan salt, if using.

Fill the glass with ice and strain the cocktail into the glass.

Garnish with the magnolia petals, then say a toast or blessing for the wonderful spring ahead. Remind yourself to love this spring and to enjoy the simple things in life.

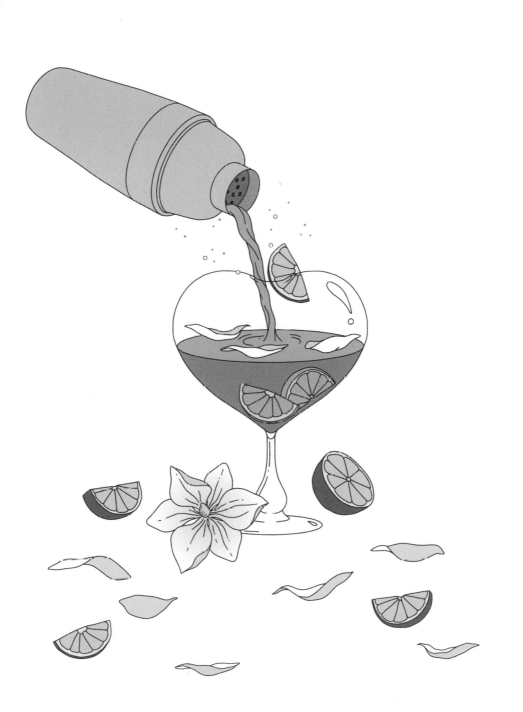

Water is our everything. It has the power not just to cleanse our body and wash away a bad day, but to bring healing, love, and to wash away the negative thoughts that we can sometimes have on repeat all day. Water represents our emotions and intuition, and serves as a reminder of our natural human state: flowing, changing, self-aware, and resilient.

Throughout history, water rituals played a part in many cultures and religions, and they still do. I was raised as an Orthodox Christian and every January we celebrated Epiphany, a holiday known as the Baptism of the Lord. The whole community would gather near a river or lake and cut holes in the ice to briefly bathe in the freezing water in commemoration of the day Jesus was baptized in the waters of the River Jordan. These holy ice baths are believed to heal the body and the mind, to bless you and cleanse you of your sins. Despite Epiphany falling on the coldest week of the year (in Siberia it was -31 to -40°F/-35 to -40°C), the community continued to participate in the tradition.

Of course, you do not have to go to these extremes to create a water ritual. Moreover, you have probably performed a water spell or taken a ritual bath hundreds of times before without even realizing it—intuitively selecting ingredients, lighting a candle, adding healing elements. A true water ritual, just like any other spell, starts with your intention: with a decision to carve some time out just for yourself, to heal your body and mind, to go deeper inward and find clarity, to take care of yourself, to bring more love into your life.

Water is a super-powerful and magical element by itself, and when you add an intention and another magical element—flowers, herbs, crystals, salt, and so on—you can create a wide range of effects: healing, manifesting, recharging, releasing. By being fully present in the water, you absorb all the qualities of the elements you are working with.

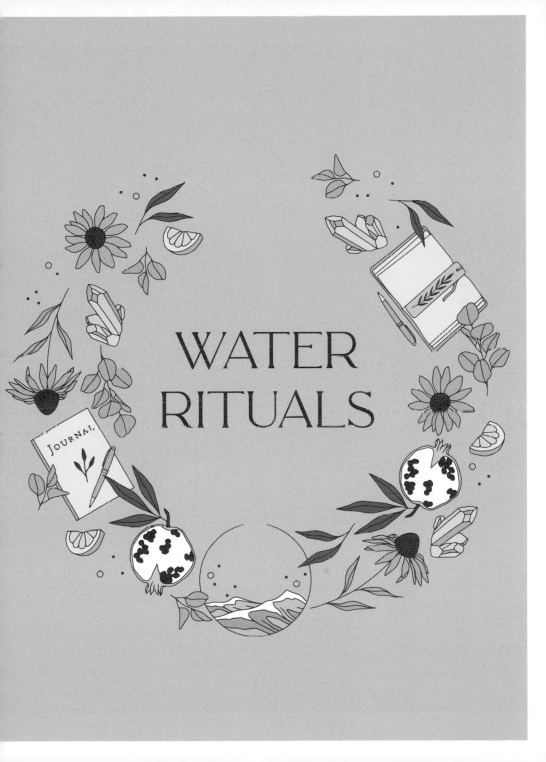

WATER
RITUALS

HERBAL BATH
FOR PROTECTION

Every time we embark on a new adventure or adopt a new path, we need protection. Protection from an evil eye, protection from the influence of others, and protection from our own negative thought patterns and fears.

So if you ever find yourself on the verge of starting something new—a career or relationship, perhaps—try this protective herbal bath. Rosemary, sage, and thyme are the most popular plants when it comes to protection spells (besides garlic). In many folk stories rosemary was used to chase demons or bad spirits away—even now, garden witches plant a rosemary bush in the garden to keep away deer or other animals, which hate the strong and earthy smell. Never underestimate the power of plants!

Ingredients:
1 cup (240 g) salt (Epsom, Dead Sea, Himalayan, etc.)
rosemary: a few sprigs of fresh, sprinkling of dried, or a few drops of essential oil
sage: a few fresh leaves, sprinkling of dried, or a few drops of essential oil
thyme: a few sprigs of fresh, sprinkling of dried, or a few drops of essential oil

Directions:
Run a hot bath and slowly add all the ingredients.

Get into the bathtub and do a few rounds of deep breathing. Once you feel relaxed, envision a protective layer covering you—an invisible bubble, protecting your mind, body, and spirit.

Relax and soak in the magic.

Witchy tip: If you ever have someone coming to your house who you are not completely comfortable with, diffuse some rosemary essential oil or burn dried rosemary before their arrival. The aura of rosemary will protect you from any negative thoughts or words.

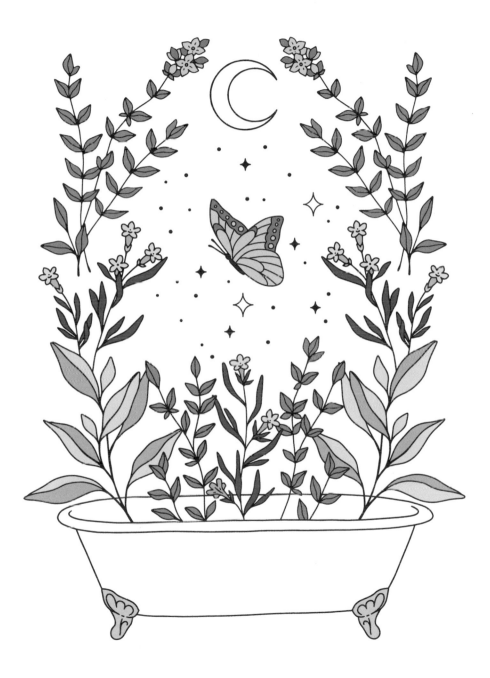

GOOD NIGHT'S SLEEP BATH

We all go through periods of poor sleep or insomnia. Sometimes the moon is to blame, sometimes the stress of work. But before reaching for sleep medicine, try a holistic approach. Reduce screen time and caffeine consumption, try yin or nidra yoga, or my favorite—chamomile tea and a warm bath an hour before sleep.

Chamomile is a gentle flower with a sweet and earthy aroma, best known for its calming properties. A simple chamomile tea or infusion can help promote restful sleep and reduce anxiety and stress. And paired with a warm bath, it makes a perfect nighttime ritual. The secret as to why baths are so beneficial is because soaking in warm water increases your body temperature and then naturally drops it. This transition stimulates the production of melatonin, which helps to make you sleepy.

Ingredients:
1–3 cups (240–720 g) Epsom salt, or any other salt with magnesium flakes
pot of chamomile tea
a few drops of lavender essential oil (optional)

Directions:
Run a hot bath and add the salt.

Pour yourself a cup of chamomile tea and add the rest to your bath along with the lavender essential oil, if using. For a mess-free bath, strain the tea before adding it to the water.

Get into the bathtub and do a few rounds of deep breathing.

Relax with your favorite music or book, if desired.

The use of chamomile has been documented as far back as Ancient Egypt. It was used to treat everything from skin rashes and digestive problems, to loss of appetite and fevers caused by malaria. Chamomile was known as a lucky flower—people would decorate their homes with it and make flower garlands or sachets. It is also a common witchy practice to plant chamomile near doors and windows, to prevent negativity from entering the house.

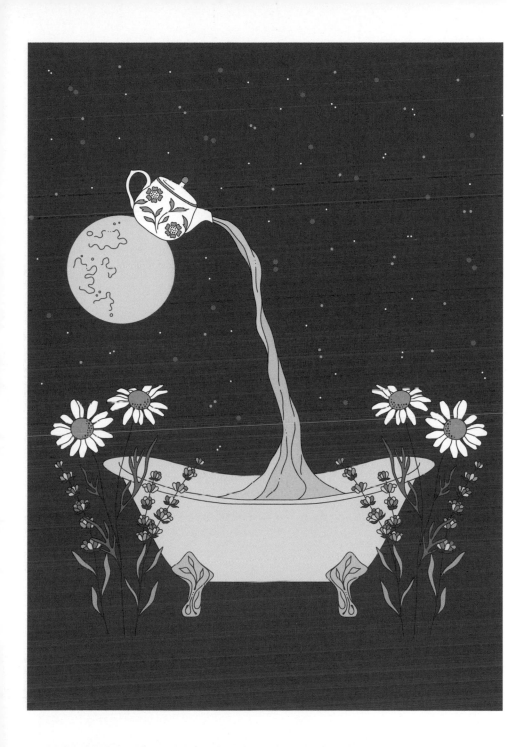

HEARTWARMING CINNAMON BATH

This cleansing bath has been inspired by one of the most magical herbs on the planet—cinnamon. Cinnamon not only has an incredible range of physical healing benefits (it helps to relieve congestion, sore throat, and stomach upsets); it also has spiritual benefits. My mom would often make me an apple pie with cinnamon, saying that this mysterious (and hard to get in Siberia) spice would help to clear any uncertainty I might have, shine light on my desires, and help me see things as they truly are. No matter where you are on your life journey, if you want to cleanse the energy around you, to raise your vibration, or get some much-needed clarity, give this cinnamon bath a try.

Ingredients:
1 cinnamon stick
1–2 cups (240–480 g) Epsom salt
1 tsp ground cinnamon

Equipment:
journal and pen

Directions:
Start this ritual by cleaning your space. If your home or work environment is cluttered and messy, you might experience brain fog. Light the cinnamon stick until embers appear, then blow them out, allowing the smoke to swirl around you. Use this smoke to cleanse the air and your aura. Do not rush this process, go slowly around your house, cleansing every single corner. Pass the smoke gently over each and every part of your body.

Run a hot bath and set your intention.

In a bowl, combine the salt with the ground cinnamon (you could also use a blender) and add the mixture to the bath. Stir the water to help distribute and dissolve it.

If you don't have any ground cinnamon, add some cinnamon tea or a few cinnamon sticks to your bath.

Get into the bathtub and do a few rounds of deep breathing.

Spend at least 15–30 minutes in the tub, allowing the cinnamon to warm your heart and soul. Once you feel relaxed, grab your journal and pen and write down everything your heart desires. Consider all the areas of your life.

The following morning, review the list and ask yourself if anything has changed since the night before. Maybe you need to add or delete an item. This is normal. Create a habit of revisiting what you want on a regular basis; consistency encourages positive change.

Witches all over the world use cinnamon in their cleansing and protection spells. The cinnamon broom is made of pine straws and cinnamon oil and is placed by the front door to create a welcoming and pleasant smell. And if you go a little further back in time, witches believed that the sweet aroma of the cinnamon broom would protect their houses from negative energies and unwanted guests.

RED CLOVER ABUNDANCE BATH

Red clover's medicine is humble and gentle. It doesn't shout, but gives freely to anyone who notices its magic. Red clover is popular among Eastern European herbalists, helping with colds, fevers, and skin conditions. It is also popular among witches and widely used in cleansing, protection, and, most importantly, abundance spells.

I love to bathe in the sweet and earthy aroma of clover. If you ever find yourself at a crossroads, hoping for that long-awaited promotion, or simply want to attract more luck and abundance into your life, try this red clover bath spell.

Ingredients:
handful of fresh red clover flowers,
  or 2–3 tbsp dried flowers
1 cup (240 g) Epsom salt
1 tbsp honey (optional)

Equipment:
journal and pen
candle (optional)

Directions:
Start by making a red clover tea. Steep the flowers in near-boiling water for at least 10–15 minutes, then strain and discard the herbs (or leave them in for extra magic).

Run a hot bath and set your intention.

Slowly and mindfully add all the ingredients to your bath. The honey will leave your skin feeling soft and moisturized, although take care if you decide to use it because the fats in the honey will make the bathtub slippery.

Get into the bathtub and do a few rounds of deep breathing.

Once you feel relaxed, use your journal to reflect on any beliefs/patterns that might be holding you back from making money. How did you feel about money growing up? What is standing between you and your dream life? Is it the belief that you are not worthy of money? That money is a source of evil? Any personal growth work can be painful and triggering, so go easy on yourself. And if there are any beliefs that don't serve you or are not in your best interest, it is time to let them go. If you wish, you can burn this piece of paper using a candle, releasing everything into the air (though please be careful).

Relax and soak in the tub for at least 20 minutes. Welcome more abundance into your life and allow good things to happen.

Some witches like to sprinkle red clover around the house, just before cleaning, to attract prosperity and good fortune; others like to make protective amulets using dried clover.

61

CEDAR FOREST BATH FOR CONFIDENCE

Confidence comes in different layers and levels—some people are confident traveling to faraway countries all by themselves, but have zero confidence when it comes to speaking up for themselves. Being confident is not just feeling secure in your mind and body; it is a deeper level of trusting yourself.

For many centuries, witches used cedar, balsam fir, and tree bark in their confidence spells. This powerful concoction was usually made in a cauldron over the open fire, and its earthy and woody smell was known to improve self-belief.

Whenever you experience a moment of doubt and need a boost of self-confidence, take a walk in a nature, gather some cedar needles, and try this forest-inspired bath. Or if you are unable to gather tree medicine, try cedarwood essential oil.

The word "confidence" comes from the Latin word fidere, which means "to trust." Therefore, having self-confidence is having trust in oneself. Trust yourself going forward. You are doing a great job.

Ingredients:
1–2 cups (240–480 g) Epsom salt
cedar needles, or a few drops of cedarwood
    essential oil

Equipment:
journal and pen

Directions:
Run a hot bath and set your intention.

Add all the ingredients to your bath.

Slowly get into the bathtub and do a few rounds of deep breathing. Close your eyes and imagine yourself in a beautiful green forest.

Once you feel relaxed, spend some time writing wonderful things about yourself in your journal. Do not hold back—this is for your eyes only. Compliment yourself. List all your accomplishments, big or small. Or perhaps write a story of how you helped someone. Or describe how it might feel to walk into a room with confidence. Simply let your fingers channel what's been stirring inside you, and envision every single word.

If there is ever a moment in your life when you begin to doubt yourself, let these pages be a reminder of how strong, capable, brave, and compassionate you are.

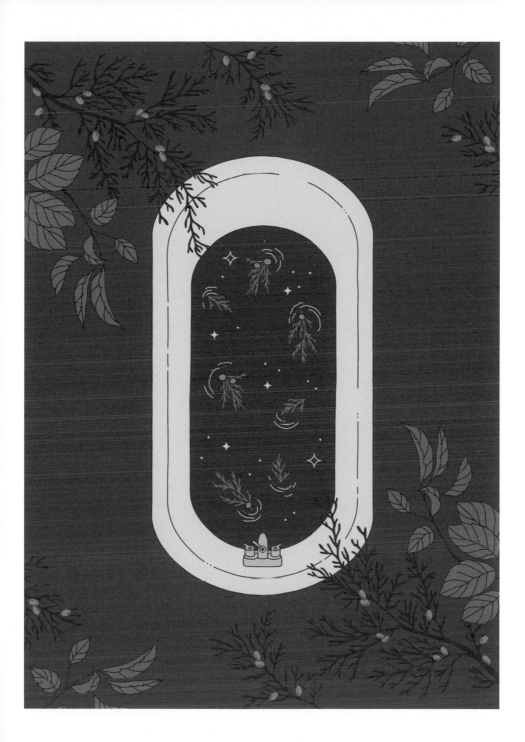

DANDELION BATH FOR INNER JOY

Dandelions are little droplets of sunshine and true heralds of spring. Their bright yellow color represents happiness, optimism, enlightenment, creativity, and sunshine. This bath is one of my favorite spring rituals, bringing light, love, and joy after a long, dark winter.

Although many people consider dandelions an annoying weed, these humble flowers can offer a variety of benefits. From tea that is known to relieve digestive issues, and vinegar that helps to relieve itchy bug bites, to dandelion salve that is incredible for dry skin. And did you know that all parts of this spring flower are edible—the leaves, flower, and even the roots? Dandelion flowers do not have any toxic look-a-likes, which makes the process of foraging fun and easy.

Ingredients:
handful of fresh dandelion flowers
1–2 cups (240–480 g) Epsom salt
a few drops of your favorite essential oil

Equipment:
journal and pen

Directions:
Start by making a dandelion salt. Mix one part dandelion flowers with two parts Epsom salt in a blender. The salt will become a beautiful pastel yellow color.

Run a hot bath and set your intention: that you want to feel excited about the next phase of your life; you want to attract more joy and laughter into your everyday life; you want to make self-love and self-care a priority— whatever it might be for you.

Slowly and mindfully add the dandelion salt and essential oil to your bath.

Get into the bathtub and do a few rounds of deep breathing.

Once you feel relaxed, reflect on how you want to feel every time you start your day. Happy? Motivated? Excited for what the day will bring? Record your feelings in your journal in the present tense, as though it is already happening: "Every morning I wake up and feel..."

If you would like to make a larger batch of salt and preserve some for the months ahead, spread the mixture on a baking sheet and bake for 10–15 minutes at a low temperature (around 200–250°F/95–120°C), stirring every few minutes. The baking will help to get rid of any moisture. Store in an airtight container, away from sunlight, for up to a year.

ENERGY CLEANSING
BATH FOR EMPATHS

I find crystals to be an especially valuable tool for empaths. They can act as a shield, protecting your aura and helping you to stay grounded when dealing with the emotions of others. And sometimes even just holding a crystal helps to center you and slow you down for a second. A particularly good crystal for empaths is black tourmaline, since no energy is strong enough to pass through its rich, dark shield. I keep one near my front door to protect the boundaries of my home, and it's always a good idea to keep one on you whenever you're out in the world, especially if you're going into an uncomfortable situation. Even if you don't consider yourself an empath, try this crystal-charged cleansing bath. You will be surprised how good you feel afterward.

Empaths feel things deeply, sense energy entering a room, and sometimes even hold on to emotions and feelings that didn't belong to them in the first place. In addition to this cleansing bath with crystals, there are lots of practices and rituals that can help empaths protect their energy field, such as visualizing a shield around themselves, and setting clear and strict boundaries.

Ingredients:

black tourmaline, or another crystal of your choice (other great crystals for empaths include black obsidian, smoky quartz, hematite, fluorite, and amethyst)

½–1 cup (100–200 g) baking soda (bicarbonate of soda) (optional)

handful of fresh rose petals (optional)

Directions:

Run a hot bath and submerge the black tourmaline crystal in the water along with the other ingredients, if using. If you are using a different crystal, make sure to check if it is water safe and, if not, place it on the edge of the bathtub.

Do a few rounds of deep breathing, relax, and let the water work its magic.

When you are ready, drain your bath, but remain in the water as it does; as the water level falls, imagine all your doubts, worries, and all the feelings that don't belong to you being washed away with it.

POMEGRANATE BATH FOR EMBRACING YOUR SHADOWS

The juicy, blood-red pomegranate, dubbed "the oldest superfood," is full of vitamins and antioxidants, and for centuries has been used to enhance general health and wellbeing. The magic of bright red pomegranate is rooted in countless myths and legends, including the Ancient Egyptian legend of Sekhmet (see next page). For Ancient Egyptians, this goddess gave inspiration to live life fiercely every day, to follow their own path, to speak their own truth, and to know their worth. In modern times, Sekhmet reminds us of our dual nature: our femininity and masculinity, our love and rage, our joy and sorrow, our light and darkness. We are complex beings, and we do not have to choose between one extreme or the other. All of it can live within us at the same time.

If there are aspects of yourself that you have been suppressing or avoiding dealing with, make yourself this dreamy bath and grab your journal. I find journaling to be a simple but effective technique when it comes to shadow work—a deep dive into your unconscious mind. Simple journal prompts can help you tap into your subconscious and shine light on even the darkest parts of your soul.

Ingredients:
1–2 cups (240–480 g) salt (Epsom, sea, Himalayan, black lava, etc.)
½ cup (120 ml) pomegranate juice and/or the seeds of 1 fresh pomegranate
a few drops of sandalwood, jasmine, frankincense, or dragon's blood essential oil
red, orange, or yellow crystals, such as ruby, tiger's eye, citrine, amber, or agate (to connect with the inner fire of Sekhmet)

Equipment:
journal and pen

Directions:

Run a hot bath and set your intention.

Mindfully add all the ingredients to the bathtub.

Place a crystal of your choice on the edge of the tub and slowly get into the water.

Once you feel relaxed and at peace, take your journal and ask yourself some difficult questions. Journal prompts are different for everyone, but here are a few examples: What does a life of self-acceptance feel and look like to you? What relationship pattern has followed you throughout your life? When are you hardest on yourself and why? How can you show more compassion to yourself? What events in your life have hurt you the most? What reminds you of these times? What part of you still remains there? When was the last time you forgave yourself? Remember, acknowledging that something exists comes from a place of strength and love for yourself.

Try not to rush; simply let your fingers channel what has been stirring inside you. Once finished, do a few rounds of deep breathing, relax, and take this quiet time for yourself.

The legend of Sekhmet
The Egyptian Sun God, Ra, wanted to punish humanity for their sins, so sent down his daughter in the form of a lioness. It was only when she reached Earth that she became Sekhmet, "The Powerful One." When Ra saw that his daughter had destroyed far more than he had ordered, he decided to calm her by pouring beer into the Nile and staining it blood-red with pomegranate juice. Sekhmet, thinking it was blood, drank the whole river down, becoming so intoxicated that she fell asleep for days. When she awoke, balance was restored.

VANILLA BATH FOR
SWEETNESS OF LIFE

Vanilla can work wonders for most foods and beverages, but it can do even more for the heart and soul. The smell of vanilla, whether it is coming from a burning candle, freshly baked vanilla cookies, or from a few drops of essential oil on the wrist, is so comforting and warm, it inspires us to love.

The idea of living a "sweet life" is the notion of living life to the fullest. This might look different from day to day—sometimes it might be not settling for less than you deserve; sometimes it is doing something that scares you; and sometimes it is taking a divine, hour-long vanilla bath.

Vanilla is a well-known aphrodisiac. It is also widely used in haircare, because of its high vitamin B and antioxidant content. But above all, vanilla is known for its uplifting power—it can provide an instant energy boost, desire, and excitement for a sweet life.

Ingredients:
1–2 cups (240–480 g) salt (Epsom, sea, Himalayan, black lava, etc.)
1 vanilla bean (if you can't find one, use a few drops of vanilla essential oil or vanilla extract instead)

Equipment:
journal and pen

Directions:
Run a hot bath and set your intention.

Before getting into the bathtub, pause and sit on the edge of the tub. Immerse your hand in the water and bless it—tell it about your dreams and goals, how you want to feel. When you are finished blessing the water, thank it for being a part of your ritual.

Get into the bathtub and do a few rounds of deep breathing.

In your journal, reflect on the things that bring you the greatest joy. In what way can you treat yourself more? What are five things you can do to bring more sweetness into your everyday life?

The following day, treat yourself to something nice.

PLANTAIN BATH SALTS TO RELEASE NEGATIVE FEELINGS AND EMOTIONS

Plantain weed grows in abundance in almost every yard and park. Yet despite its name, it is actually one of the best healing and edible plants. Not to be confused with the plantain fruit, this shy plant offers a variety of benefits and has been used since Ancient Greek times. It is wonderful for the skin, reducing inflammation and promoting wound healing. In summer, the young leaves can be eaten fresh in salads.

In witchcraft, plantain is used in healing balms, protection amulets, and to add strength to and empower spells or rituals. Adding plantain leaves to your bath salts will not only nourish your skin, but will enhance the cleansing properties of salt, helping you to release any stagnant or negative feelings that you might have been holding on to.

Ingredients:
1–2 cups (240–480 g) Epsom salt
handful of fresh plantain leaves
1–2 tsp dried lavender buds or a few
   drops of lavender essential oil (optional)

Equipment:
journal and pen

Directions:
Combine the salt, plantain leaves, and lavender in a blender.

Run a hot bath and set your intention.

Slowly and mindfully get into the bathtub and sprinkle in some of the salt.

Once you feel relaxed, ask yourself if there are any emotions or feelings that no longer serve you. If there is something, it is likely holding you back from achieving your full potential. I know how uncomfortable and intense it might feel to get out of what is familiar and safe, so be gentle with yourself. It is ok to admit that something no longer works. It is ok to change and let those emotions go.

If you would like to make a larger batch of salt and preserve some for the months ahead, spread the mixture on a baking tray and bake for 10–15 minutes at a low temperature (around 200–250°F/95–120°C), stirring every few minutes. The baking will help to get rid of any moisture. Store in an airtight container, away from sunlight, for up to a year.

HIBISCUS BATH
FOR CLAIRVOYANCE

Exotic and seductive hibiscus comes in many unusual colors and variations, yet is almost always associated with love, devotion, passion, vitality, glory, and beauty. Hibiscus has been (and still is) widely used for divination rituals—it was burned as incense, and there is an old tradition of placing hibiscus flower petals in a bowl filled with water. It was believed that by gazing at the flowers swimming gently in the water, one could see the future. This bath was inspired by this mystical and intriguing ritual. It might not show you the future, but sometimes we don't need to see the future to know that everything will be all right. Sometimes we just need to remind ourselves how capable and strong and passionate we are, and that everything that we wish for will find its way to us. So let this bath be an opportunity to trust and love yourself more.

Ingredients:
handful of fresh or dried hibiscus flowers (if you can't find hibiscus flowers, use hibiscus powder or a pot of hibiscus tea instead)
1 cup (240 g) pink Himalayan salt (optional)
1 tablespoon honey (optional)

Equipment:
pen and paper

Directions:
Run a hot bath and set your intention.

Slowly and mindfully add all the ingredients to your bath.

Get into the bathtub and do a few rounds of deep breathing.

Spend at least 15–30 minutes soaking in the tub. Gaze at the surface of the water and focus on the feeling of the warm water against your skin. Allow all thoughts to disappear.

Using the pen and paper, write a letter to your future self—it could be one year into the future, five, or even ten. I usually choose a one-year time frame since it is easier to envision your goals and make a plan.

Consider different areas of your life. What lessons have you learned? What goals have you achieved? Do you take enough care of yourself? How do you show love for yourself? Once you are done, fold the letter and date it, then keep it in a safe place until needed. Reading a letter like this can have such a cathartic and profound effect. It can show you how much you have grown; how much closer you are to your goals than you might think; and how there is absolutely no reason to not trust yourself or the Universe.

Relax and enjoy this precious time you have carved for yourself.

Hibiscus flowers have been used for centuries as a powerful aphrodisiac. There are stories of Ancient Egyptians drinking hibiscus tea to induce feelings of lust, while in China hibiscus flowers were given to both women and men as a symbol of success.

OATMEAL BATH TO OPEN
THE DOOR FOR HEALING

One of the best-known benefits of oatmeal is its ability to cleanse, hydrate, and nourish the skin. That is why oatmeal baths are one of my favorite self-care rituals. Clear your schedule and make yourself the dreamiest, milkiest bath ever.

Oats are widely used in different rituals and spells. Some say that oats "open the door that allows healing to take place." Oats are believed to create a sense of peace, supporting emotional wellbeing.

Ingredients:
1 cup (90 g) oats (instant, quick cook, regular rolled oats, etc.)
1–2 cups (240–480 g) salt (Epsom, Dead Sea, Himalayan, etc.)
a few drops of your favorite essential oil
1–2 cups (240–480 ml) milk of your choice (optional)
handful of fresh or dried flowers (rose, calendula, jasmine, etc.) (optional)

Directions:
Start by grinding the oats into a fine powder, using a blender or coffee grinder. The powder should be fine enough to evenly disperse in the bath and make it milky.

Run a hot bath and set your intention.

While the water is still running, slowly and mindfully add all the ingredients to the bathtub.

Get into the tub and do a few rounds of deep breathing.

Admire the beautiful milky bath you have created. Relax and soak in the magic.

GROUNDING DIANTHUS BATH

If you ever find yourself distracted, anxious, or daydreaming, these could be signs that you are not grounded. Grounding is the practice of bringing balance into the body through connection to Mother Nature. There is no greater medicine than Mother Nature. She has the power to heal and rejuvenate our body and soul, helping us to get in touch with our true self and allowing our body and mind to access our true talents and hidden powers.

Start your grounding ritual by spending some quality time outside, breathing deeply. And when you are ready to come back inside, take this root-chakra-inspired dianthus bath. The root chakra, or Muladhara, is located at the base of the spine. It provides a base or foundation for life, helps you feel grounded, and gives you the ability to withstand challenges. Your root chakra is also responsible for your sense of security and stability.

Ingredients:
3 cups (720 g) Epsom salt
handful of fresh red dianthus flowers
(red is the color of the root chakra)

Directions:
Run a hot bath and set your intention

Slowly and mindfully add the ingredients to your bath.

Get into the bathtub and do a few rounds of deep breathing.

Relax and soak in the magic

> *Other grounding rituals include:*
> - *Walking barefoot, imagining long roots extending from the soles of your feet.*
> - *Gardening (preferably without gloves).*
> - *Eating root vegetables.*
> - *Forest bathing or hiking.*
> - *Swimming in rivers and lakes.*
> - *Spending at least 15 to 30 minutes outside each day.*

ECHINACEA BATH FOR VITALITY

Echinacea was considered (and still is by a lot of herbalists) the number-one plant for vitality and health, especially during the long, cold winter months to treat cold and flu.

A simple echinacea bath is an excellent way to utilize its healing powers, not to mention its benefits for the skin. Take this bath on a cold winter night to bring more love and light into your life. Or when you have a cold, try combining echinacea and ginger for a detoxifying bath.

It's not just homemade cold remedies that are made with this magnificent plant—many medicines sold in drug stores contain echinacea, from cough syrups and immune-boosting teas, to nasal sprays and bath soaks.

Ingredients:
pot of echinacea tea
pot of ginger tea or a handful of freshly grated root ginger
1–2 cups (240–480 g) Epsom salt
½ cup (100 g) baking soda (bicarbonate of soda)

Equipment:
journal and pen (optional)

Directions:
Run a hot bath and set your intention.

Brew the echinacea and ginger teas, then pour yourself a cup (of either or both!) and add the rest to your bath.

Add the remaining ingredients and slowly get into the bathtub. Do a few rounds of deep breathing.

Spend at least 20–30 minutes soaking in the bath, allowing the echinacea to work her magic.

At the end of your ritual bath, think about how you can bring more wellness into your daily life. Perhaps reflect on your habits, or consider how you can prioritize your health—both mental and physical—on a daily basis. You can record your thoughts in your journal, if desired.

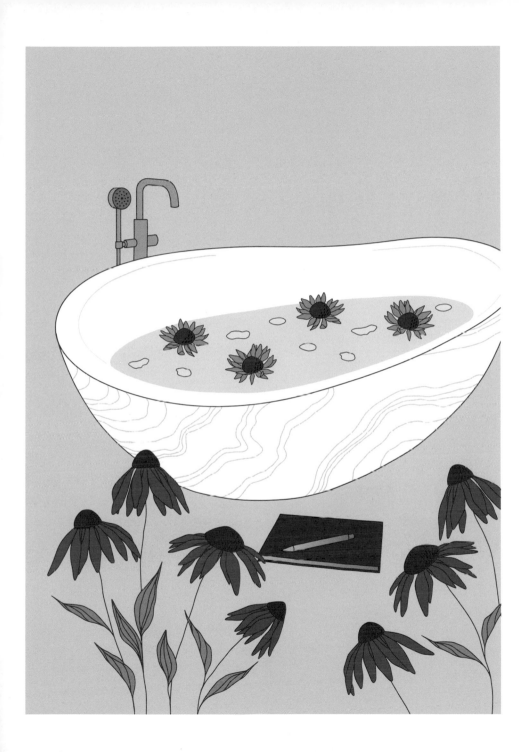

YARROW SALT BATH TO CAST A CIRCLE

Like all other magical flowers, yarrow's benefits mirror its spiritual properties. Its magic is deeply rooted in mythology. The full name of common yarrow is *Achillea millefolium*—the name taken from Achilles, the Ancient Greek hero who was immortal and invincible except for his heel. The name was linked to the hero's myth because of its reputation as a powerful wound healer. Yarrow is believed to banish melancholy from your body and help ground you and re-establish your foundations. It is also perfect for casting circles—creating a safe and protected space for any magic work.

I like to cast a circle when there is a big question burning inside my chest and I want to create a safe, completely neutral space in which I can explore my thoughts and desires. So if you ever find yourself coming back to the same question over and over again, try casting a circle with yarrow. Let her protect and shelter you from negative influences and self-doubt, and remind you how invincible, invulnerable, and loved you are.

Ingredients:
¼ cup (15 g) fresh or dried yarrow flowers
½ cup (120 g) Epsom salt, sea salt, or pink Himalayan salt
a few drops of your favorite essential oil (optional)

Equipment:
journal and pen

Directions:
Start by mixing your yarrow flowers and salt in a blender.

If you are working with fresh flowers, spread the mixture on a baking sheet to dry, or bake it at a low temperature (around 200–250°F/95–120°C) for 15–30 minutes, stirring frequently. By drying the salt, you are ensuring that it will stay fresh for longer and help prevent clumps forming.

Run a hot bath and set your intention.

Get into the bathtub and sprinkle the yarrow salt in a circle around you to create the safest, most comforting, and supportive space. Add the essential oil, if using.

Once you feel relaxed, ask yourself that big, scary, exciting question. There is nothing to fear. You are supported, protected, and loved. Take a deep breath and let your fingers channel your inner wisdom onto the pages of your journal.

When you are finished, close the circle. Thank the water, salt, and flowers for being a part of your ritual. And, most importantly, say a few words of appreciation and gratitude to yourself—for taking time out of your busy schedule and making yourself a priority.

Casting circles means different things to different people—some like to draw a pentagram on the ground, some like to envision an invisible bubble around them, and some like to create a circle made of salt. Casting a circle is simply creating a mental space in which you can be your true self, not holding anything back; where you shine your light without fear or judgment, and where you love yourself fully and unconditionally.

PASSIONFLOWER BATH TO WASH AWAY HURTFUL WORDS

We have all been victims of the hurtful words of others. Sometimes we can brush them off easily, but other times they stick. We repeat them in our head, having an invisible, and what feels like an eternal, dialogue. And they just keep on hurting us. Passionflower is a great ally when it comes to relieving anxiety, helping to stop that mental chatter and find peace of mind.

Always remember who you are. And that no one in the world can take that from you. So always choose to show up as yourself. Shine your light no matter what. And choose to not give power to any words or actions that don't serve your greatest good.

Ingredients:
handful of fresh passionflowers (if you can't find passionflowers, use a pot of passionflower tea or 2 drops of tincture)
1 cup (240 g) black salt (optional)
a few drops of your favorite essential oil (optional)

Directions:
Run a hot bath and set your intention.

Slowly and mindfully add all the ingredients to your bath, then get into the tub.

Soak for at least 15–25 minutes, allowing the passionflower to calm and nurture your soul.

When you are ready, drain your bath, but remain in the water as it does. As the water level falls, imagine all the negative feelings being washed away, and all the hurtful words going down the drain.

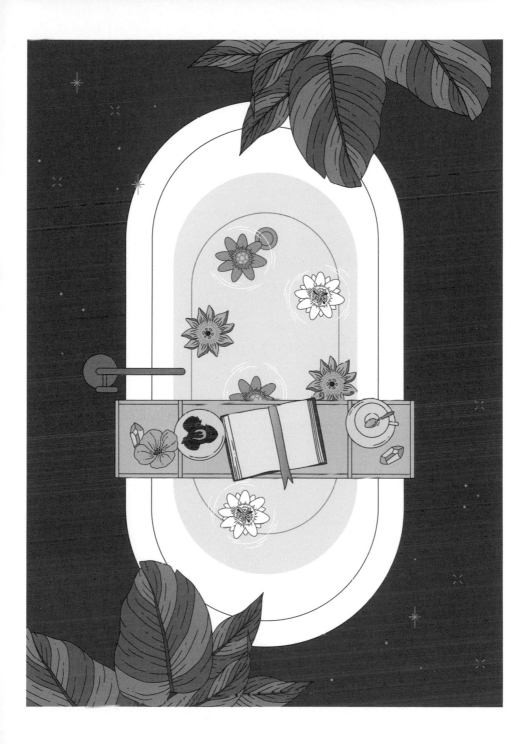

HEALING MILKY BATH

For the last few years, I have been fascinated with ancient goddesses. The simple realization that all goddesses—from brave Artemis to sensual Freya—are alive within me brought so much peace, courage, and excitement into my heart, and helped me to tap in to all that knowledge.

This dreamy bath has been inspired by Isis, Egyptian goddess of fertility, magic, and healing, mother of the Egyptian Kings, and a witch. Isis represents the deep and ancient mystery of the feminine ability to heal, create, and bring forth life; when her son, Horus, was wounded, she healed him with the power of her milk.

The main ingredient of this luxurious bath is coconut milk, though you can use any milk of your choice. Remember, the most important thing is your intention.

Ingredients:
1–3 cups (240–720 g) salt (Epsom, sea, Himalayan, etc.)
5 cups (1.2 l) coconut milk (or milk of your choice)
handful of fresh or dried rose petals
rose quartz crystal (optional)

Directions:
Begin by turning off your phone, and perhaps bring a book, cup of tea, or glass of wine to the bath with you.

Run a hot bath, dim the lights, and slowly add all the ingredients to your bath (please take care, because the fats in the milk can make your bathtub slippery).

Get into the bathtub and do a few rounds of deep breathing. Allow the milk to soothe your aching heart and the salty water to cleanse and wash away all the negative thoughts.

If you have a rose quartz, place it on your heart to promote healing and self-love. Say out loud: "I love myself deeply and fully." Relax and enjoy this precious time that you have carved out for your beautiful self.

If you want to make your own coconut milk, try this simple recipe. It only takes a few minutes. Blend 4 cups (960 ml) hot water with 2–2½ cups (80–120 g) shredded unsweetened coconut until thick and creamy. Strain the mixture through cheesecloth or a fine-mesh strainer, making sure to squeeze and twist out every drop. Store in a 32 oz (950 ml) jar with a lid, in the refrigerator, and use within three days. Shake well before using.

BORAGE AND CUCUMBER FOOT BATH FOR A FRESH START

Never underestimate the power of a good foot bath. Soaking your feet relieves aches and pains, stimulates circulation, alleviates stress, and promotes relaxation and a good night's sleep. According to Chinese medicine, your entire body is connected to your feet, so it makes sense that caring for your feet can bring health and comfort to your whole body.

This foot bath was inspired by long summer nights and azure borage flowers. Every garden witch knows to plant borage in her garden because it attracts pollinators and repels certain harmful bugs. Its beautiful blue flowers and leaves are completely edible—and taste just like cucumber. Borage is known for helping to fight indecisiveness and doubt, bringing determination, courage, and self-confidence. There is even an old saying: "I, Borage, always bring courage." Try this foot bath to help you unwind after a long day and to leave all your worries behind, so you can start fresh the next day.

Ingredients:
1 cup (240 g) Epsom salt
½ cup (100 g) baking soda (bicarbonate of soda)
1 cucumber, sliced
handful of fresh borage flowers or a few drops of borage oil

Directions:
Add warm water to a large bowl (make sure it is not super hot).

Add all the ingredients and find a comfortable seated position—on a couch or chair with a pillow behind your lower back, perhaps.

Soak your feet in the bowl for at least 20 minutes.

If you have any cucumbers left, make a cucumber face mask. Cut the cucumber into very thin slices and apply to your face and eyes. Cucumber is full of vitamins and minerals and can help soothe inflammation, lessen redness, and prevent blemishes.

LEMON FOOT BATH FOR ENERGY AND MOTIVATION

We all go through periods of lethargy, burnout, apathy, or laziness. And that is ok. Everything in the Universe strives for balance. If there is time for hard and intense work, there is time for complete rest and unproductiveness. Try to navigate these moments without judgment. Stay there as long as you need to, allowing yourself to rest and recuperate fully. Then when you are ready, get out of your head and just move your body: dance, go for a walk, experience a change in scenery. And go get yourself some lemons and oranges.

Citrus fruits—lemons, oranges, grapefruits, etc.—are some of the most powerful tools for energy and inspiration, evoking our senses and clearing brain fog. Try this lemon foot bath (you could also use it in a full bath) for an instant boost of energy and motivation.

Ingredients:
1 cup (240 g) Epsom salt
½ cup (100 g) baking soda (bicarbonate of soda)
1 lemon, sliced, or a few drops of lemon essential oil

Equipment:
journal and pen

Directions:
Add warm water to a large bowl (make sure it is not super hot).

Add all the ingredients and find a comfortable seated position—on a couch or chair with a pillow behind your lower back, perhaps.

Soak your feet in the bowl for at least 20 minutes.

After this energizing foot bath, create a list of inspiring ideas in your journal: opportunities, collaborations, new projects, trips... You could even make a vision board! Do everything you can to remain energized and inspired to keep the momentum going.

The smell of lemon can boost production of serotonin, a hormone that makes you feel happy, and reduce levels of the stress hormone. When you feel your energy levels dropping or need a little pick-me-up, before grabbing a coffee or energy drink, cut a lemon (or any other citrus fruit) in half and inhale the smell for 30 seconds or more. Or try citrus essential oil on your wrist. You will be surprised how much better you feel.

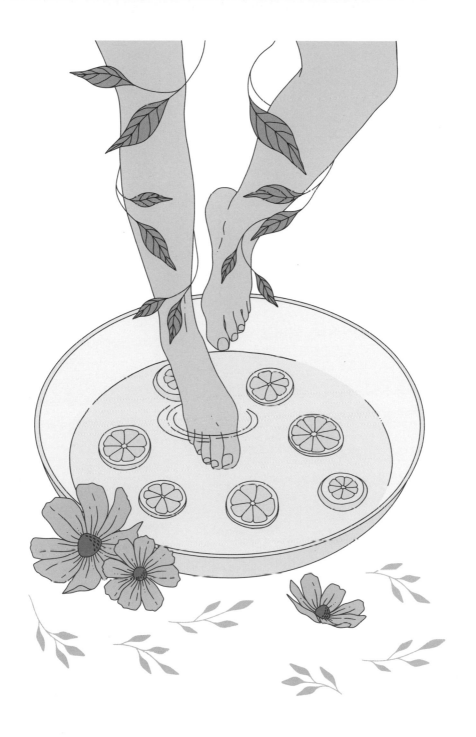

HORSETAIL HAIR RINSE TO REMOVE CREATIVE BLOCKS

In many witchy traditions it is believed that hair absorbs our energy, our thoughts, and our vibrations, good and bad—this is perhaps why it feels so good to cut our hair after big life changes. If you are going through some creative blocks, have had a stressful day at work, or an emotional argument with your partner, you don't have to go to the extreme of cutting your beautiful hair. Try a hair rinse with horsetail (also known as shave grass). It is believed that this simple plant was around long before humankind walked the Earth, and it is packed with vitamins and plant collagen—exactly what your hair needs.

Another ingredient in this hair rinse, apple cider vinegar, is absolutely magical for your hair and scalp. Its cleansing properties will not only remove all negative energy and impurities, but also help strengthen the hair.

Ingredients:
¼ cup (10 g) dried horsetail
1 tbsp dried lavender (optional)
1 tbsp dried rosemary (optional)
1 tbsp dried rose petals (optional)
16 fl oz (450 ml) just-boiled water
2–4 tsp apple cider vinegar

Equipment:
16 oz (450 ml) glass jar
journal and pen

Directions:
Steep all the dried herbs in the just-boiled water for 10–15 minutes. Strain the liquid into the jar, discarding the herbs (or leave them in for extra magic), then leave to cool before adding the apple cider vinegar.

While this wonderful potion is cooling down, find a comfortable seat and write down all the obstacles you see in your path¬—both internal and external blocks. Try not to rush this process, but just let your heart go.

Once you have finished journaling, shower as normal and, after shampooing and conditioning your hair, slowly pour the rinse over your hair evenly, working it into your scalp, feeling all your worries melting away. Let it sit for a couple of minutes before rinsing out.

In the morning, review the list of obstacles and see how you feel and if anything has changed since the night before. Perhaps some of the blocks don't seem like such a big deal anymore. Or perhaps this powerful duo of horsetail and vinegar has helped you shine a light on your problems and you will find a solution in a new and surprising place.

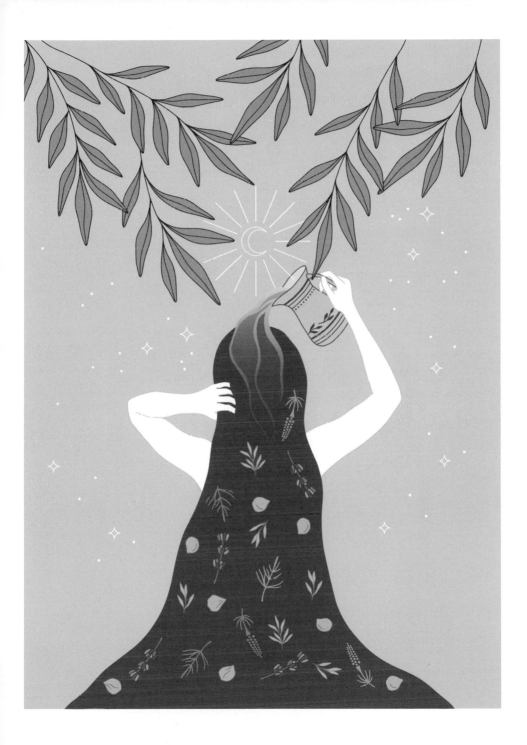

BAY LEAF ELIXIR FOR PROPHETIC DREAMS AND LUXURIOUS HAIR

Bay leaves were probably the most used herb in our house—from making tea to preparing delicious stews and soups. It is one of the few plants that increases its flavor and smell after being dried, so it's not surprising it has been used for centuries to stimulate appetite. In addition to being one of the most aromatic herbs, bay leaf is exceptional for hair care (due to its antibacterial properties) and could be very helpful for cleansing and detoxifying your scalp, especially if you have dandruff or oily hair.

Sometimes, when I'm at a crossroads, I like to do "bay leaf nights." I start by cleansing my aura with the smoke of bay leaf. And as the evening progresses, I make the bay leaf elixir for my hair, filling every corner of the house with its exciting and cleansing aroma. I take a slow shower, washing away all my worries, and as I get ready for bed, I ask the questions that have brought me to this crossroads. The magic happens at night, as bay leaf is known to bring clarity and attract prophetic dreams.

Ingredients:
½ cup whole dried bay leaves
4 cups (960 ml) water

Equipment:
32 oz (950 ml) jar with lid/bottle
  with spray nozzle for storage
journal and pen

Directions:

In a medium saucepan, bring the bay leaves and water to a boil. Reduce the heat and let it simmer for at least 20 minutes. Once the aroma is strong, turn off the heat and let it cool. Discard the bay leaves and pour the elixir into a jar or bottle for storage; I prefer a bottle with a spray nozzle for easy application. The elixir will keep in the fridge for up to a week.

Take a slow shower. Perhaps put on a relaxing playlist to set the mood. Before shampooing your hair, apply a generous amount of bay leaf elixir onto damp hair. Leave it on for 5–7 minutes before shampooing.

Before going to bed that night, take a dry bay leaf and write on it the goal, situation, or vision you need clarity on. Put it under your pillow. The minute you wake up in the morning, write down everything that came to you during the night in your journal. What did you see? How did it feel? Sometimes you receive a clear answer, sometimes you receive symbols and signs to investigate. Take the time to analyze the message you have been given. Within it is the answer.

Other ways you can use bay leaves:
- *Use the smoke of a bay leaf to cleanse your space and your aura.*
- *Carry a bay leaf with you (I keep one in the car) to ward off negative energy.*
- *Use a bay leaf for a letting go spell. Simply write what you wish to release on a bay leaf and light it (make sure you have a bowl of water handy, and watch out for spitting). As you watch the things you wrote go up in flames, imagine them being released and disappearing from your life.*

FORGIVENESS BATH TEA

I find that forgiving yourself is the hardest form of forgiveness—no one in the world judges us more than we judge ourselves. Not even a superhuman can keep up with our unrealistically high expectations. Go easy on yourself. Forgive yourself for your mistakes because, in reality, there is no such thing as a mistake. There is only knowledge, wisdom, and experience. Your forgiveness journey is unique to you, and it does not have to look a certain way. Just do what feels right to you. Forgiveness frees us to live in the present, which is where life happens.

Green tea is known for its wide range of benefits, from supporting metabolic health to helping to lower cholesterol levels. Let this simple green tea bath nurture and support your soul.

Tea is one of the most compassionate and tender plants. In the witchy community, tea is believed to promote emotional healing and forgiveness. We drink tea at family celebrations and make tea for our friends when they go through rough times.

Ingredients:
pot of green tea
1–2 cups (240–480 g) Epsom salt

Equipment:
pen and paper

Directions:
Run a hot bath and set your intention.

Pour yourself a cup of green tea and add the rest to your bath.

Add the salt, slowly get into the bathtub, and do a few rounds of deep breathing.

Once you feel relaxed, write a letter to someone you would like to forgive. If you need to forgive yourself, write a letter to yourself. Take as much time as you need to write the letter. If writing a personal letter is too painful, simply write: "I forgive you. I release you. I am setting myself free." You can keep the letter, tear it into small pieces, burn it, or bury it. Do what feels right to you.

Relax. Breathe. Feel yourself become lighter. And let all your worries go down the drain as you pull the plug.

STINGING NETTLE TEA TO REMOVE NEGATIVE THOUGHTS

If there is one plant that immediately takes me back to my childhood, it is the stinging nettle. It grew in abundance near our house, and I would come home covered in nettle stings from head to toe. But my mom used to say it was good for me—that not only would it be a natural boost for my immune system, but that the burning sensation was the negativity leaving my body.

Witches associate nettles with a protective and mothering nature. It is believed that nettle has the power to shift and transform our thoughts, to nurture the soul and heal the body, supporting and encouraging us, just like a mother. If you ever find yourself having repetitive negative thoughts, constantly playing in the background in your head, try this simple nettle tea rinse (and boost your hair's health at the same time).

Herbalists love nettle for its nutrient content—it is absolutely packed with vitamins, minerals, and amino acids. A simple cup of nettle tea could be a great remedy for many different concerns, and especially hair health. It is known to help with hair breakage, hair loss, and regeneration of hair follicles.

Ingredients:
¼ cup fresh or 2–3 tsp dried nettle leaves
16 fl oz (450 ml) just-boiled water

Equipment:
pen and paper
16 oz (450 ml) glass jar

Directions:
Use the pen and paper to write down a negative thought that keeps appearing in your head. On the opposite side of the paper, transform it into something positive by writing a thought you want to replace it with. Steep the nettle leaves in the just-boiled water, then submerge your paper in the tea. Allow the tea to brew for at least 10–15 minutes.

Strain the tea into the jar (or you could leave the herbs and paper in for extra magic). Leave to cool.

At the end of a shower or bath, close your eyes and slowly pour the jar of tea over your head. Let it all go down the drain, every single negative thought.

Massage the nettle tea into your scalp, let it sit for a couple of minutes, then rinse it out.

AMETHYST SHOWER
FOR EMOTIONAL BALANCE

Water is so powerful and magical that it can turn anything into a ritual. This amethyst shower is one such ritual—a perfect and quick way to restore balance to your life and release all the pressure you put on yourself. You might know amethyst as "the all-purpose stone," perfect for everyday spells. But it is also one of the most powerful crystals when it comes to balancing the emotions. It is used as a protective stone, helping to relieve stress, anxiety, fatigue, and exhaustion.

When taking a shower, visualize it washing away all your stress, anxiety, and negative thoughts. Concentrate on the feeling of the water upon your skin. Breathe deep. Let it all go down the drain, and welcome light and balance.

Ingredients:
amethyst crystal

Equipment:
journal and pen

Directions:
Start by making amethyst water. Leave an amethyst (or any other crystal of your choice) in water overnight. The water will absorb all the magical properties of the crystal.

Turn on some soothing music to help you set the calming mood.

Shower as you normally would, but this time take the crystal-charged water into the shower with you (remove the crystal first) and whisper your intentions to it. Then pour it slowly over your head, letting the water run down your body. Crystal water works miracles, and you will be surprised how good you feel after this quick shower.

After the shower, sit down with your journal and pen. Split a blank page into two columns. In the first column, write a list of things that are overwhelming you or that you are overindulging in. In the second column, write what you would like to see more of in your life. When your lists are complete, review them without judgment. Try to find the good in the bad, and the bad in the good. Be gentle with yourself. Recognize that everything on your list has its time and place in your life. This step is not about punishing yourself for bad habits, but to see things closely and clearly. It is about finding your strengths and identifying areas for growth.

The next morning, do one thing from the second column and skip one thing from the first column. See how it feels. Life is all about making mistakes, learning, growing, and balancing.

If you do not have an amethyst crystal, try rose quartz, clear quartz, citrine, or tiger's eye instead. These are just as magical as amethyst, and they are also water safe.

EUCALYPTUS SHOWER TO SHARPEN THOUGHTS AND REMOVE THE INFLUENCE OF OTHERS

Eucalyptus is known for its menthol-like scent and a long list of health benefits, from relieving muscle pain to treating nasal congestion. Eucalyptus naturally calms the mind and soothes irrational anxieties.

My favorite way to bring more of the magic of this incredible plant into everyday life is a simple eucalyptus shower. Water infused with the properties of eucalyptus has the power to wash away a bad day, negative thoughts, unkind words, and any bad influences, and the steam released by the oils of the eucalyptus plant will fill your entire bathroom with a stress-relieving aroma. It is also good in the morning to promote alertness and clarity of thought.

In the witchy community, eucalyptus is known for its cleansing and protective properties. There are stories of witches cleaning their floors with eucalyptus-infused water after unwanted guests, or burning leaves to cleanse their aura of the influence of others.

Ingredients:
a few sprigs of fresh eucalyptus
natural twine or rubber band

Directions:
Tie the eucalyptus stems together with natural twine or a rubber band and attach them to the shower head. Ideally, position the eucalyptus so it is not directly under the water stream. If you do not have fresh eucalyptus, try diffusing eucalyptus oil while showering.

Turn the water on and let it run for a minute, allowing the shower stall or room to fill with steam, and with the aroma and magic of eucalyptus.

Shower as you normally would, but this time breathe slowly and envision the water as white light showering you in its cleansing, soothing vibrations. Wash away every negative thought. You may even say out loud: "I am free of the negative influences of others. I see things as they truly are, I speak my own truth..."

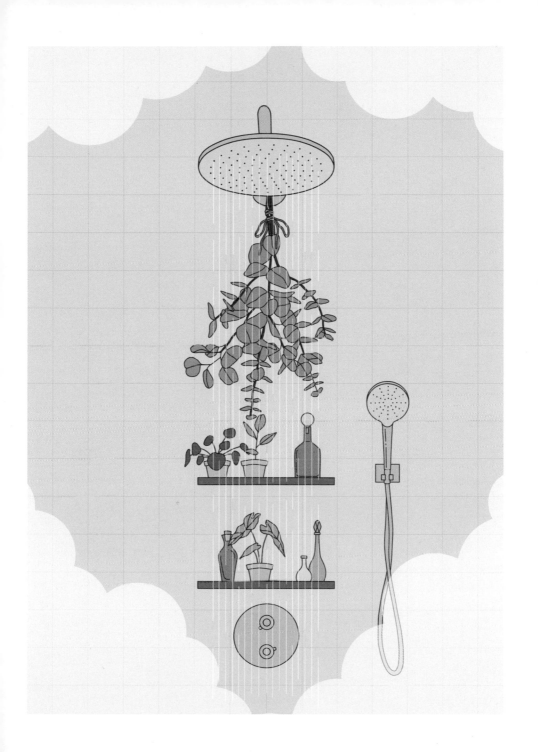

Home and body rituals could be any act of love or compassion that we show to ourselves. Sometimes it is simply laying on the couch, ignoring our to-do list, and allowing body and mind to fully rest and recuperate. And sometimes it is an enchanting full moon candle spell.

More often than not, we don't give enough credit to these rituals. We judge everything by productivity and results. But these simple rituals provide us with an opportunity to slow down and take better care of ourselves. They serve as a reminder that it is our own selves with whom we need to fall deeply in love in order to connect with the outside world in a harmonious way. Because love doesn't just come from outside of us. It begins within.

This chapter includes magical potions that can help you take care of yourself and your body, cleanse the energy in your house, invite more confidence into your life, and promote healing. Some of these herbal potions take weeks to make—but that just serves as a reminder that you are worthy of your own time, care, attention, and all the flowers in the world. You are worthy of loving yourself fully, exactly as you are.

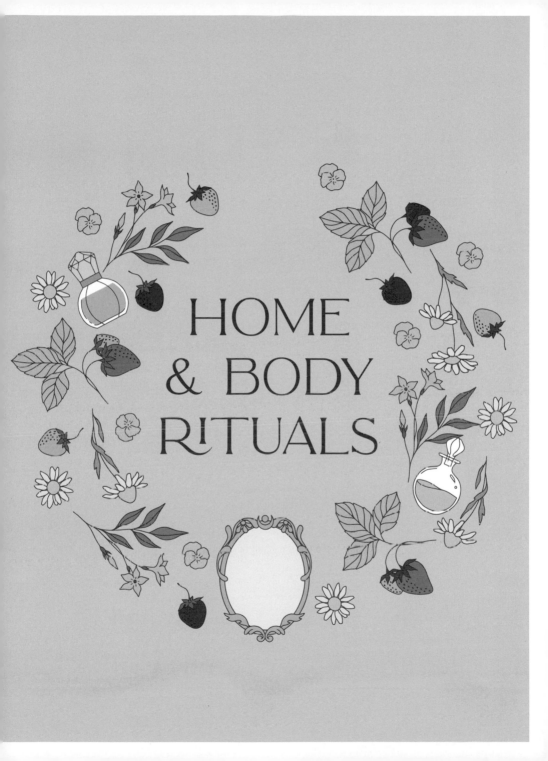

HOME
& BODY
RITUALS

HONEY JAR FOR MANIFESTING SPELL

Witches love using sweeteners in their spells and rituals. The fluid nature of honey and syrups is meant to help us achieve what our heart truly desires, with fewer obstacle and barriers. This spell was inspired by Freya, the Norse goddess of love and war. Freya teaches us about self-awareness, self-worth, and self-love. She sees the beauty in everyone and everything. And she reminds us to enjoy ourselves by singing and dancing and making love. So learn from Freya—be present in your body and experience the emotions and sensations felt only by human beings. Freya's essence is represented by honey, the main component of this spell.

Freya, the Norse goddess of love and war, is associated with sex, lust, beauty, witchcraft, fertility, and abundance. She is a seeker of pleasure, thrills, and passion. Some believe she only cares for the chaos of desire, but modern pagans and witches know that Freya is much more than a lover or a passing nightmare. She is a powerful, ancient goddess. She is a warrior queen, a shapeshifter, and a wild and untamed force of nature.

Ingredients:
small jar of honey
herbs, crystals, or other elements
(see directions)

Equipment:
pen and paper
1 small mason jar with a metal lid
1 small votive candle

Directions:
Sit down with a pen and paper and write down what your heart desires. It could be anything: I want to love myself more; I want to be a published author by this time next year; I want to meet my soulmate. Whatever the desire, be as specific as possible.

Once finished, roll up the paper and place it inside the jar. You may also choose to add some herbs, crystals, or other elements. This is an intuitive part of the spell and depends on what kind of intention you are working with. If you are asking for love, you could include rose quartz or rose petals. If you are looking for financial abundance, perhaps a dollar bill, a coin, or some basil. Listen to your inner voice. Pour the honey over the contents of the jar until it is filled. Fasten the lid tightly.

Once finished, place a votive candle on top of the lid, and ask Freya for guidance and support. Let the candle seal your spell by dripping wax down the sides of the jar.

Keep the honey jar by your bed or on your altar, if you have one. Keep it for as long as you feel connected and aligned with everything you wrote, or until your wish comes true.

CALENDULA INFUSED
OIL FOR INNER SUN

If any flower embodies the warm essence and glow of the sun, it's calendula. The flowers quite literally resemble the sun, and symbolize warmth, optimism, and inner joy. Calendula is also one of the best-known medicinal plants—famous for hydrating and nourishing skin. Plus, its anti-inflammatory and antioxidant properties not only help to repair any damage, but protect your skin in the future.

This easy-to-make calendula oil is especially wonderful during the long winter months, when our skin feels dry and the sun keeps hiding from us. Use it on your hair, nails, elbows, or on any part of the body that needs a little extra love and sunshine.

Every time you apply this sunny potion, take a minute and think (or journal) about the ways in which you can bring more joy and happiness into your everyday life. Ask yourself how you would shine your light if no one was looking. Let the calendula nourish your skin, and let your positive thoughts inspire and reassure you.

Ingredients:
1 cup (40 g) fresh or ½ cup (20 g) dried
   calendula flowers
1 cup (240 ml) apricot kernel oil, or any other oil
   of your choice (almond, argan, rosehip seed,
   and jojoba oils are all wonderful alternatives)
½ tsp vitamin E oil (optional)

Equipment:
2 x 8 oz (225 ml) glass jars with lid
cheesecloth (or other piece of fabric) or a
   fine-mesh strainer, for straining

Directions:
Fill a jar three-quarters full with calendula flowers. Add the oil of your choice until the jar is full, or until the herbs are covered by at least 1 inch (2.5 cm). The flowers expand as they soak in the oil, so make sure they stay covered.

Leave to infuse for 4–6 weeks. Since the calendula flowers resemble the sun, I like to solar infuse this magical potion by leaving the jar outside or on a sunny windowsill. Another approach suggests protecting the oil and flowers from UV light, in which case place the jar in a paper bag before leaving in a sunny spot.

Give the jar a good shake every other day or whenever you walk by it.

After 4–6 weeks, strain the oil through cheesecloth or a fine-mesh strainer, into a clean glass jar. Discard the flowers. Add the vitamin E oil, if desired; its antioxidant properties will help prolong the shelf life of the oil.

Store in a cool, dark place, to use within a year.

JASMINE DREAM PILLOW

Lucid dreaming is being aware that you're dreaming and, in most cases, being able to control the dream's storyline and environment. Sounds pretty amazing, right? Lucid dreaming also has therapeutic effects, from reducing anxiety and nightmares, to boosting creativity and problem-solving skills. It is a great opportunity to first visualize and then execute your plans and goals. Some people even use lucid dreaming to find creative and unusual ways to solve complex and real-life problems. Finding solutions to your problems or seeing your goals fulfilled (even in your dreams) can be a very positive and encouraging experience, filling your heart with confidence and love.

If you would like to try to stimulate these visionary dreams, I highly recommend working with jasmine flowers. Jasmine has a calming effect on the nervous system, but is also known to increase psychic abilities and enhance lucid dreaming. And one of the easiest ways of incorporating this incredible flower into your sleeping ritual is by making a dream pillow.

Ingredients:
handful of dried jasmine flowers
handful of dried lavender
handful of dried chamomile flowers (optional)
handful of dried rose petals (optional)
handful of dried lemon balm (optional)

Equipment:
large muslin drawstring bag

Directions:
Start by mixing together the herbs and flowers of your choice.

Place the mix in the muslin drawstring bag and fasten tightly.

Keep the bag next to your bed. Before drifting off to sleep, try to envision your goals, or the situation you need clarity on, and see where the dream pillow takes you.

Although many people agree that lucid dreaming can be very beneficial, it might interrupt your sleep, and it is definitely not for everyone. I highly recommend reading more about consciousness dreaming and perhaps exploring different techniques. And do not put pressure on yourself if you can't figure it all out right from the start.

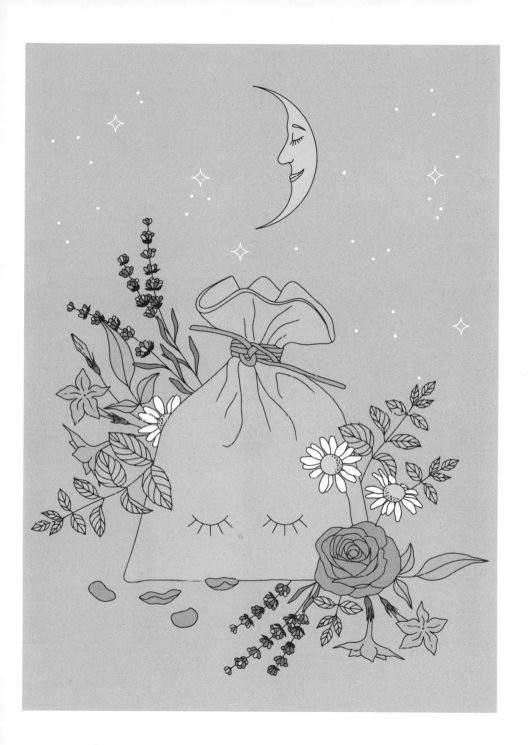

NUTMEG SPELL FOR SOLO TRAVELING

Many of us are familiar with the warm and almost intoxicating aroma of nutmeg, which can bring back good memories. In witchcraft, nutmeg has been widely used in travel, protection, health, and good luck spells. It is believed that carrying a whole nutmeg in the pocket will help to ensure good luck while traveling.

When I was younger, I used to love traveling solo. Nothing would ever scare or bore me. But as I grew older, I forgot how to enjoy and love my own company. I would feel bored at times, anxious, or even guilty for taking time off. So for the last year or so, I have been unpacking these issues, and a nutmeg has been my loyal companion. Not only does it shield you from any troubles, it warms your heart and reminds you how incredibly interesting and wonderful you are, how you deserve the world at your feet. But if you don't fancy carrying a nutmeg with you at all times, try this simple candle ritual before heading out on your adventure.

Ingredients:
pinch of nutmeg

Equipment:
1 small candle (a simple container
   or pillar candle works best)
journal and pen (optional)

Directions:

Sprinkle the nutmeg over the top of your candle. When working with such a powerful and potent spice, always remember that a little goes a long way. A pinch is all you need.

When you are ready to book your solo trip, light the candle and place it next to you. Let the delicious aroma of protective nutmeg accompany you right from the beginning of your adventure. Or if you're not quite ready to book and simply want to plan your trip, grab your journal and pen and describe what your perfect solo trip would look like. Record as many details as possible—how you would dress, whether you would sleep in or wake up with the sun, how you would visit all the places your friends would not have wanted to go to, how flexible you are going to be...

And when you are done planning your amazing trip, before blowing out the candle, say: "I enjoy the pleasure of my own company. I am worthy of all the wonderful things in the world." And say it like you mean it!

The history of nutmeg has not always been happy and peaceful. During the seventeenth century, the Dutch fought a long and bloody war against the Bandanese people in Southeast Asia in an attempt to gain control over the islanders' spice and nutmeg production (until the mid-nineteenth century, the Banda Islands were the only source of the spice). Some even call nutmeg the "bloody spice" as a result of the war.

NURTURING ARNICA BALM

Arnica is one of the most famous homeopathic herbs. It is known to help with muscle aches and strains, to reduce inflammation, and to soothe joint pain. It is especially popular in Europe, particularly in Germany, where it is believed they created over 100 medicinal uses for arnica—treating everything from heart disease to bruises.

The beautiful yellow flowers of arnica are usually associated with the pagan holiday of Midsummer. Arnica was also used as an offering to ensure an abundant and successful harvest. And there are stories of arnica being used by pagans as a spiritual protective barrier—it was said to have been planted around corn and wheat fields to prevent the "spirit of the wolf" or "Corn Wolf" escaping the field before the grain was ready to be harvested. It was believed that the "wolf" added his strength to the coming harvest.

If you ever want to create a protective barrier around yourself, and nurture your beautiful skin at the same time, try making this incredible balm.

Ingredients:
½ cup (20 g) fresh or ¼ cup (10 g) dried arnica flowers
1 cup (240 ml) olive oil
1 cup (140 g) beeswax pellets (feel free to substitute with soy)
½ tsp vitamin E oil (optional)

Equipment:
heatproof bowl (glass or ceramic) or a canning jar
cheesecloth (or other piece of fabric) or a fine-mesh strainer, for straining
4 oz jar with lid (or two 2 oz metal tins, so you can easily carry the balm with you)

Directions:

Fill a jar three-quarters full with arnica flowers. Add the olive oil until the jar is full, or until the flowers are covered by at least 1 inch (2.5 cm). As the flowers soak in the oil they will expand, so you want to make sure they stay covered.

Leave to infuse for 2–4 weeks.

After this, strain the oil through cheesecloth or a fine-mesh strainer into a clean heatproof bowl, and discard the flowers.

Add the beeswax to the bowl.

At the same time, put about 1 inch (2.5 cm) water into a saucepan over a low heat and place the bowl in the saucepan to create a double boiler. Stir constantly until all the ingredients have melted. Add the vitamin E oil, if desired; the antioxidant properties of the vitamin E will help prolong the shelf life of the balm.

While warm, pour the balm into the container(s) of your choice and allow to cool at room temperature for at least 24 hours.

Store in a cool, dark place for up to a year.

Balms are a little different from salves. They tend to be harder and thicker, containing a higher ratio of beeswax (1:1 ratio wax to oil). Salves have a softer consistency, and a lower ratio of beeswax (1:4 ratio of wax to oil). But both balms and salves have the same goal—to make you and your beautiful skin feel better.

To ensure your salves and balms have the desired consistency, as soon as you have melted the ingredients in the double boiler, dip a clean spoon into the mixture and place it in the fridge to cool. If the mixture is too hard, add a little more oil. If it is too soft, add a little more beeswax.

DAISY SALVE TO SOOTHE A BRUISED HEART

Daisies are a symbol of purity, love, transformation, new beginnings, renewal, and healing of a bruised heart. And since the spiritual properties of plants are always intertwined with their medicinal uses, it's no surprise that daisies were also used for centuries to treat swelling, irritated skin, and especially bruises. Some even say that the phrase "oopsy-daisy" came about not only because it was used to encourage a child who had fallen, but also because a daisy would be used to treat a child's bruise.

So if you ever need support in your healing journey, or want to nurture your aching heart and skin, try making this daisy salve. Apply it to your heart area and other parts of your body that might benefit from the healing and renewal properties of daisies, and repeat: "I will come out of the darkness even stronger than before. Every ending offers me the opportunity for a beautiful new beginning. My happiness comes from within. I allow myself to move slowly through this healing journey and take my time. I am strong. I am resilient. I am whole. I am worthy. I am enough. I am loved."

Ingredients:
½ cup fresh (20 g) or ¼ cup (10 g) dried daisy flowers
1 cup (240 ml) olive oil
¼ cup (35 g) beeswax pellets (feel free to substitute with soy)
½ tsp vitamin E oil (optional)

Equipment:
heatproof bowl (glass or ceramic) or a canning jar
cheesecloth (or other piece of fabric) or a fine-mesh strainer, for straining
4 oz (115 ml) jar with lid (or two 2 oz/60 ml metal tins, so you can easily carry the salve with you)

continued on next page

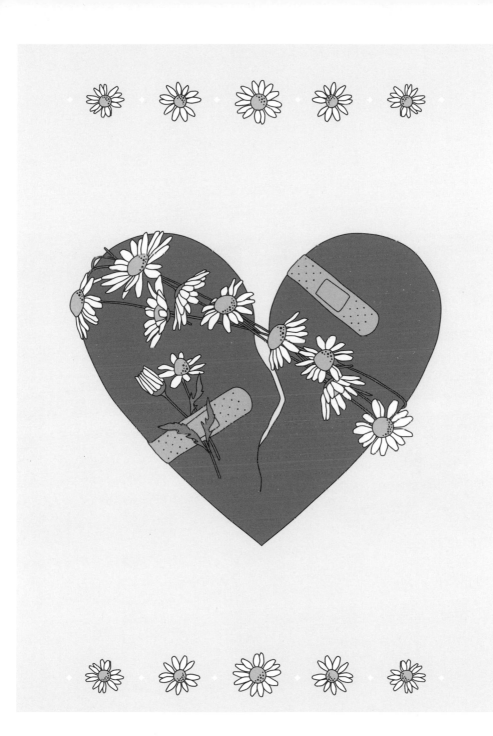

DAISY SALVE FOR A BRUISED HEART

There are so many legends and myths about daisies. In Celtic legend, there is a heartbreaking story about God sprinkling daisies over the earth whenever a child died, to cheer and nurture the parents. In Norse mythology, a daisy was the sacred flower of Freya, the goddess of love and war, and was associated with love and fertility. And in Roman legend, there is a story about Vertumnus, the god of seasons and gardens, who fell in love with a nymph by the name of Belides, chasing her constantly; to escape his pursuits, she turned herself into a daisy.

Directions:

Fill a jar three-quarters full with daisy flowers. Add the olive oil until the jar is full, or until the flowers are covered by at least 1 inch (2.5 cm). As the flowers soak in the oil they will expand, so you want to make sure they stay covered.

Leave to infuse for 2–4 weeks.

After this, strain the oil through cheesecloth or a fine-mesh strainer into a clean heatproof bowl, and discard the flowers.

Add the beeswax to the bowl.

At the same time, put about 1 inch (2.5 cm) water into a saucepan over a low heat and place the bowl in the saucepan to create a double boiler. Stir constantly until all the ingredients have melted. Add the vitamin E oil, if desired; the antioxidant properties of the vitamin E will help prolong the shelf life of the balm.

While warm, pour the salve into the container(s) of your choice and allow to cool at room temperature for at least 24 hours.

Store in a cool, dark place for up to a year.

EDIBLE STRAWBERRY SCRUB
TO INVOKE THE GODDESS

Strawberries are associated with Venus, the goddess of love. Their beautiful red color and heart shape are symbols of love, fertility, beauty, pleasure, confidence, and self-esteem; and, of course, awareness of your self-worth and value. Modern herbalists use this magical fruit in prenatal care, and in heart tonics and teas to help lower cholesterol and keep the heart healthy and strong. Also, strawberries have a high vitamin C content, making them perfect for skincare remedies.

If you ever need a gentle reminder that you are a real-life goddess and deserve the best the world has to offer, try making this luxurious strawberry scrub.

An old witchy spell says that if you break a strawberry in half and share it with your love interest, you will fall madly in love with each other, and your love will be sweet and sensual, just like the strawberry itself. So why not bite into a strawberry, then eat the second half yourself, and fall in love with yourself over and over again.

Ingredients:
1 cup (200 g) granulated or coarse white sugar
¼ cup (50 g) coconut oil
½ cup (80 g) fresh strawberries
dash of honey (optional)

Equipment:
16 oz (450 ml) glass jar with lid

Directions:
Combine the sugar, oil, and strawberries in a bowl until the mixture looks creamy and delicious. You could also use a food processor or blender. Store this edible scrub in a jar in the fridge until needed, and use within 2–3 days.

Once you feel ready to treat yourself, take a nice long bath or shower. Apply this scrub gently to your damp skin. Work from the feet up and over the entire body.

Go very slowly and let the strawberries stimulate your senses. Allow yourself to feel like a goddess. Focus on the texture of the sugar and strawberries against your skin. As you apply the scrub, whisper compliments to your beautiful, hardworking body. Tell it how much you love it. And thank it for carrying you through this life.

Rinse off with warm water. Please be careful because the oil from the scrub can make the bathtub slippery; be sure to rinse and wipe it down afterward.

The following day, treat yourself to something nice.

MINT LIP BALM FOR COMMUNICATION

Mint can be very helpful with reducing anxiety, relieving headaches and nausea, and aiding digestion. And as for its magical properties, it is widely used for protection and cleansing rituals, but also to attract good fortune and increase sexual desire. In fact the magic of mint is so potent that even without performing any spells or rituals, the aroma sharpens our thoughts and energies and excites us.

This simple lip balm is my go-to before interactions with new people, especially if I'm feeling nervous. The mint is energizing, waking up every cell in my brain, and helps with both psychic and verbal communication. It adds strength and confidence to my words. If you ever need a boost of boldness and self-love before leaving the house, try this invigorating lip balm.

Mint is one of the easiest herbs to grow. It comes back year after year, asking nothing in return. And there are hundreds of different varieties, from chocolate mint to apple mint, all of them fragrant and delicious. Try planting some yourself—but be warned that it spreads fast!

Ingredients:
1 tbsp beeswax pellets
4 tbsp coconut oil (sweet almond, jojoba, olive, and apricot kernel oils are all good alternatives)
1 tbsp shea butter
10 drops peppermint essential oil

Equipment:
heatproof bowl (glass or ceramic) or a canning jar
3–4 oz (90–115 ml) metal tin

Directions:
Combine the beeswax, oil, and shea butter in the heatproof bowl or jar. At the same time, put about 1 inch (2.5 cm) water into a saucepan over a low heat and place the bowl in the saucepan to create a double boiler. Stir constantly until all the ingredients have melted.

Add the drops of essential oil and stir.

While warm, pour the balm into the metal tin and allow to cool at room temperature for at least 24 hours.

Enjoy soft lips. Kiss often. And use within a year.

TULSI FACE EMULSION FOR SELF-ESTEEM BOOST

Tulsi, also known as tulasi or holy basil, is one of the most mystical plants and has exceptionally rare qualities and benefits, from physical healing to nourishing the soul. Even though the tulsi plant can be grown everywhere nowadays, and is found in stores worldwide, this ancient plant has to be treated with respect and gratitude. Every time you are lucky enough to be in the presence of tulsi, make sure to thank her for being a part of your day.

In the Sanskrit language, tulasi means "the incomparable one." Tulsi is a sacred plant in Hindu tradition and is believed to be an avatar of the goddess Lakshmi. It has been a part of Eastern culture for the last 5,000 years or so. Some refer to it as "the elixir of life," "the queen of herbs," or "mother medicine of nature."

Ingredients:
2 tbsp oats (instant, quick cooking, regular rolled oats, etc.)
1 cup (25 g) fresh tulsi leaves or 2 tbsp tulsi powder
1 tbsp milk of your choice

Directions:
Start by grinding the oats into a very fine powder using a blender or coffee grinder.

If you are working with fresh tulsi leaves, blend them until they form a smooth paste.

Combine the oats, tulsi paste or powder, the milk, and a few drops of water, and mix together thoroughly.

Apply the emulsion evenly to your face and neck and leave it on your skin for 10–15 minutes.

Rinse it off with warm water. And don't forget to tell your reflection how beautiful you are!

SALT BOWL FOR A WORKPLACE

When it comes to cleansing, there is nothing more powerful than salt. Salt crystals absorb all negativity in the air.

I like to make salt bowls when other cleansing rituals are not accessible or convenient, such as in a workplace. If your colleagues are not into witchy things, they probably wouldn't appreciate you cleansing your desk with the smoke of cinnamon or mugwort. So if you ever want to quietly cleanse your space and aura without anyone noticing, try making this simple salt bowl.

I am often asked if you can make a salt cleansing bowl and leave it secretly on someone else's desk or in someone's house, to cleanse their space. However, as the intention is the most important aspect of any spell or ritual, without the intention of the person concerned, this would not work. More importantly, no ritual or spell should ever be performed without consent, no matter how wonderful or selfless your own intention is. If you feel as though a friend needs help or might benefit from a cleansing ritual, have an honest conversation and perhaps offer to make a cleansing salt bowl (or perform any other cleansing ritual) for them.

Ingredients:
1 cup (240 g) salt (sea salt, Himalayan, black lava, etc.)
a few drops of essential oil (optional)
a few sprigs of herbs or flower petals (optional)

Directions:
Put the salt into a bowl.

You could add some essential oils, herbs, or flower petals at this point, if desired. This is a creative and intuitive part of the ritual, so do what feels right to you. Some like to add another powerful cleansing element, such as eucalyptus, cinnamon, or sage. Others like to bring more joy and happiness to their workplace and so add citrus or calendula. Or create an aura of love by adding roses.

As you mix everything together, set your intention. Perhaps: "May this salt cleanse the energy of my space and protect me from negativity..."

Place your salt bowl in your preferred location in your workspace or home and leave it overnight. Or for a deeper cleanse, leave it in place for two days.

Once finished, discard the salt. You don't want to eat it or cook with it, since it has absorbed all the negativity.

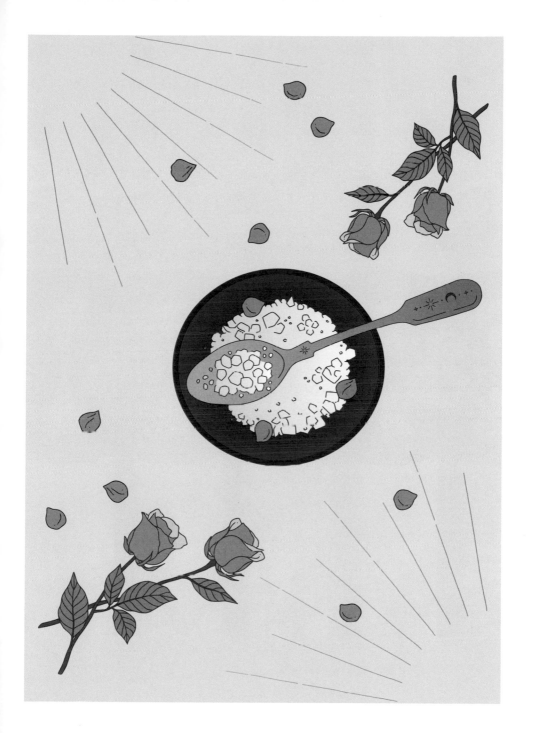

HERBAL WAND FOR SPELL CASTING

A herbal wand, just like any other magic wand, serves two main purposes: to help you focus and direct your energy, and to empower you.

This herbal wand features mugwort. It is one of the first plants to appear in the spring, and the one I am always most excited for. Her young shoots are edible and delicious, and I love making mugwort tea to help ease my menstrual cramps and aid digestion.

Use this herbal wand to enhance your self-love spells and rituals, or simply use it to cleanse the energy around you and invite in more love and light. And remember: your magic wand doesn't cast the spells. You do. You are the caster, and you hold the ultimate power.

Mugwort is known as a lunar herb, and has a deep connection to the Divine Feminine. Mugwort holds the gentle energy of receiving. It helps us to see things through intuition and feelings, rather than logic, and helps us tap into our body and inner wisdom. And it encourages love in all her forms, from romantic endeavors to deep and profound self-love.

Ingredients:
handful of fresh mugwort sprigs
handful of fresh lavender sprigs (optional)
handful of fresh rosemary sprigs (optional)
handful of fresh sage sprigs (optional)
handful of fresh thyme sprigs (optional)

Equipment:
string or twine

Directions:
Gather the herbs of your choice into a bundle.

Using string or twine, tie the herbs at the base with a secure knot to create your wand.

Wrap the string up toward the top of the wand, then return the string to the bottom in the same manner, creating a crisscross pattern. Ensure that you are crossing tightly enough that nothing gets loose, but not so tight that the herbs are crushed.

Trim off any excess pieces of herb or string.

Hang your wand upside down and let it dry for at least a week.

Once your wand is completely dry, light one end and allow it to burn for just a second.

Set your intention or affirmation for the ritual. It could be: "I am love. I am cleansing my place of negativity and self-pity and inviting more love and exuberance. May the smoke of mugwort destroy my negative thought patterns and bring more compassion and love for myself..." Then blow out the flame.

Move slowly around your house, passing the smoke gently over each part of your body. As you do so, repeat your intention or affirmation. Cast the spell with your words and let the mugwort support you.

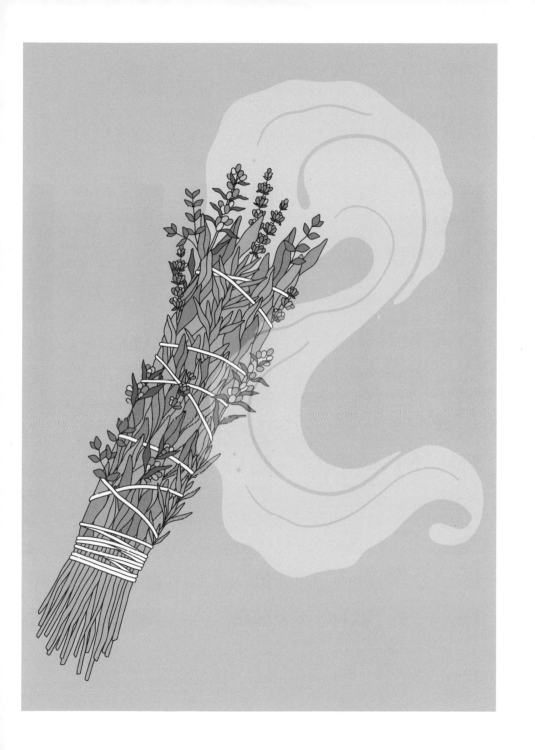

CANDLE ATTRACTION SPELL

Candles spells have been around for thousands of years—probably as long as the candle itself. One of the reasons candle magic is so popular among witches is because it is driven by the element of fire—of transformation and rebirth. Candle spells can be used for healing, releasing, manifesting, attracting, and, of course, bringing more self-love into your life.

This attraction spell simply requires a candle and something to carve with, so give it a try. I like to perform attraction spells during the waxing moon, when the moon is growing from new to full. The energy around us is building, and it is all about attracting opportunities and bringing light into our lives.

I remember performing my first candle spell when I was a broke student. I managed to buy a bright green candle, then carved dollar signs all over it and spent half the night gazing at the flame. I did not win the lottery the next day, nor did money appear out of nowhere on my doorstep, but I did find a good and well-paid job that month, which was all I wanted.

Ingredients:
a few drops of your favorite oil (olive, almond, coconut, sunflower, etc.)

Equipment:
journal and pen (optional)
small taper candle and holder
carving knife, small scissors, or toothpick

Directions:
Start this spell by thinking about what you would like to attract. What type of energy? What circumstances? What opportunities? You may also journal about it.

Once you are clear on what you would like to attract at this moment, take your candle and carve words or symbols into it that represent your desires. Depending on the softness of the candle you work with, you could use a carving knife, small scissors, or even a toothpick. Try not to rush this process. Be mindful of every stroke you carve.

Once you have finished carving, rub a few drops of your favorite oil over the entire candle to seal the spell. Some call this "dressing up the candle," while some believe you are making a psychic connection between yourself and the candle.

Place the candle in the holder and light it. Sit with it for some time and gaze at the flame. Visualize your desires as if they have already happened. Allow good things to come into your life.

HOW TO MAKE YOUR OWN TAPER CANDLES

Making your own candles—especially taper candles—in the old-fashioned way may sound like a complicated and messy process. But it is incredibly rewarding at the same time, and puts you in an almost meditative state, as you dip candles in wax and cold water again and again.

Ingredients:
3 lb (1.3 kg) beeswax pellets, or any other wax of your choice

Equipment:
large pot
deep and narrow heatproof container
90–100-inch (around 2.5 m) braided
   candle wick
hex nuts, to act as a weight to keep the candles
   straight while you dip them in the wax
deep jar of cold water
parchment paper, for drying

Directions:
Grab your large pot and fill it with 3–4 inches (7 ½–10 cm) of water. Place on the stove over medium heat.

Fill the heatproof container with beeswax pellets and carefully place it into the large pot to create a double boiler.

As the wax begins to melt, keep adding more pellets until the wax is at least 6–7 inches (15–18 cm) deep.

While the wax is melting, cut four wicks (or however many candles you are making) to 25 inches (64 cm) in length. Tie a hex nut to both ends of each wick.

As soon as the wax is melted, fold the wicks in half, with the nuts still tied at both ends. Slowly lower the nut ends into the wax, then lift them out and allow the excess wax to drip back into the pot.

Next, dip the wicks into the jar of cold water.

Dip back into the hot wax, then back into the cold water. Repeat about 8–12 times. At this point the candles should have enough weight and will stay straight on their own, so you can cut the weights off at the bottom. Make sure to cut as close to the nuts as possible.

Continue dipping your candles back and forth, between the wax and the water, until you have reached the desired diameter of the candle.

Allow the candles to cool off and harden. You can hang them or place them on parchment paper for at least a couple of hours.

Trim the wicks if needed. You can also trim the bottom of the candle to give it a flat rather than rounded shape.

Your beautiful candles are ready! Use them in your spells and rituals, decorate your bathroom with them, or gift them to friends.

LAVENDER LOVE MIST

Lavender is one of the best-known plants in the world. People were aware of its healing properties since ancient times and used it to treat infections (especially bacterial), different skin conditions, and insomnia. It was also used in cosmetic products and, of course, fragrances.

Nowadays, lavender is most famous for its incredible ability to soothe the nerves, ease anxiety, and clear the mind. A simple lavender spray is a great way to bring more love and serenity into your home. Spray it around yourself after a long workday to destress. Mist your aura to clear the mind before meditation. Spray it around your house after an argument to cleanse the energy. I like to spray it on my bedsheets as I iron them, to promote a restful night's sleep. The list is endless.

Ingredients:
1 cup (240 ml) distilled water
15–20 drops lavender essential oil
1 tbsp vodka/rubbing alcohol/witch hazel
   (alcohol helps to dissolve the oil in the
   solution and preserve the scent)
dried sprig of lavender (optional)

Equipment:
8 oz (225 ml) glass spray bottle

Directions:
Slowly and mindfully add all the liquid ingredients to the bottle.

Add the lavender sprig to the bottle for extra magic, if desired.

Shake well and use the spray as needed.

Lavender is a symbol of purity, devotion, serenity, grace, and calmness. Its purple color is associated with the crown chakra, higher purpose, awakening, and awareness.

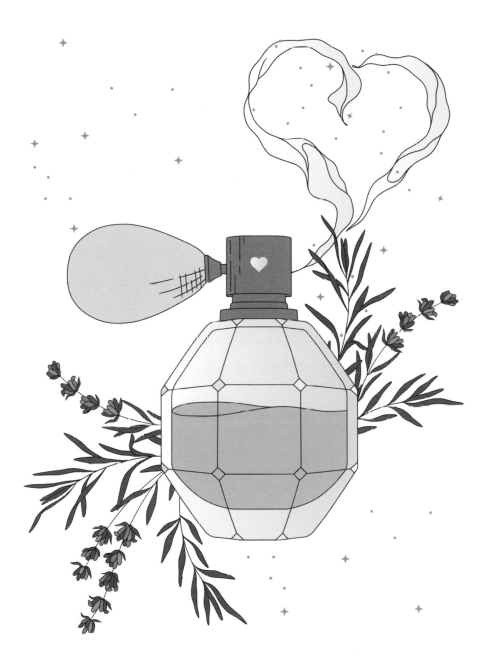

TURMERIC FACE MASK
TO BRIGHTEN THE DAY

Turmeric is one of the most scientifically studied spices, known worldwide for its ability to heal inflammation from the inside out—it is truly magical. Turmeric is associated with purity and abundance. And because of its bright yellow color, it is believed to hold the masculine energy of the sun. If you feel you have been living on the moon side lately, going through transformations, spiritual awakenings, resting, and sleeping a lot, you might enjoy working with this plant. It brings sun to your moon, creativity to your transformation, form to your dreams, and energy to your day. Neither energy is superior to the other, but in order to live a harmonious life, a balance between the two must be reached.

Use this simple turmeric mask to brighten your day and your skin, and to restore balance, if needed.

Turmeric is a great beauty product. It has been known to help with pigmentation, acne, and even wrinkles. There is a long history of brides in India using turmeric as a full body scrub and face mask to brighten their skin before the wedding.

Ingredients:
½ cup (120 g) plain yogurt
pinch of turmeric powder
dash of honey (optional)

Directions:
In a small bowl, mix together the yogurt, turmeric, and honey. Remember to use only a pinch of turmeric. This bright spice can leave stains on your skin, clothes, and towels. If you are not sure about the consistency of your mask, or if you feel you have added too much turmeric, do a simple skin patch test. Apply a thin layer on your arm and leave for 1 minute before rinsing off. If you notice no discoloration after 1 minute, leave on for another 4–5 minutes and check again.

Cleanse your face and apply the mask evenly all over. As you do so, say: "I am the sun to my own moon." Embrace your dualities, your ups and downs, your productivity and rest, your laughter and tears. It is everything that makes you YOU—so unique and special.

Leave the mask on for 10–15 minutes.

Rinse off, then apply a moisturizer, and enjoy your perfect glowing skin.

ALOE MASK FOR EXTRA GLOW

Aloe is one of the most medicinally valuable houseplants; some traditions even refer to aloe as the "immortality plant" for its incredible healing properties, and because of its ability to regenerate and heal itself. Aloe has antioxidant and antibacterial properties, and so many different skin benefits—it can help with irritation, acne, blemishes, and wound healing. It is also known as the original sunburn soother.

A face mask is one of hundreds of potions you can make with this nourishing plant. Use it to moisturize your skin after a long day at the beach, or for extra glow before an important day. And remember that your intention is one of the most important elements—put as much emotion and conviction into it as you can, embodying your affirmations and feeling them with every cell of your body.

Despite the harsh, dry climate of Siberia, our aloe plant thrived. Any time I would scrape my knee or burn my finger trying to help in the kitchen, my mom would break one of the aloe leaves, scoop the gel out, and apply it to the wound. It worked every time.

Ingredients:
aloe gel from 1 leaf, or 1 cup (240 ml) organic aloe juice
a few drops of freshly squeezed lemon juice
dash of honey (optional)

Equipment:
8 oz (225 ml) glass jar with lid

Directions:
In a bowl, combine the aloe gel or juice with the lemon and honey.

Apply the mask to your face and neck. As you do so, with every stroke you make, say a positive affirmation to set the tone for your day: "My skin and my entire body is glowing with health;" "I am open to new opportunities;" "No challenge is too great for me;" "I attract things that bring me joy, I am resilient, I attract success;" "A thousand invisible hands support my journey;" "I am courageous." Say it out loud, and really mean it.

Leave the mask on for 15–20 minutes, then rinse off and apply a moisturizer.

Store the leftover mask in a jar in the fridge for up to two weeks. You can also freeze the mixture in an ice cube tray for a cooling mask. Simply roll the cube all over your face in the morning to both de-puff and nourish your skin at the same time.

OREGANO VINEGAR
FOR AN AURA OF LOVE

It is believed that oregano contains ten times more antioxidants than other common herbs—it is that potent and powerful! Traditionally, oregano is associated with love, luck, protection, communication, and travel. An oregano plant by the house was believed to protect against evil spirits and negativity. Burning oregano was thought to open channels of communication and make conversations more flowing and interesting. Oregano was even used in spells to help forget past lovers. It infuses everything with an aura of love.

If you ever find yourself stuck or uninspired, having nightmares, feeling pessimistic, and wanting to get rid of stagnant energy from your home, try making this oregano-infused cleaning vinegar. Not only will it help you cleanse your house of negativity, dust, and dirt, it will also breathe the aura of love into your home. It is not recommended to use cleansing vinegars on natural stone, such as marble or granite, or unfinished wood, so take care.

Ingredients:
handful of fresh oregano
peel of 1 lemon
2 cups (480 ml) white vinegar
2 cups (480 ml) water

Equipment:
16 oz (450 ml) glass jar with lid
cheesecloth (or other piece of fabric)
  or a fine-mesh strainer, for straining
8 oz (225 ml) glass spray bottle(s)

Directions:

Place the oregano and lemon peel in the jar and fill it with vinegar. Make sure to cover all the ingredients completely.

Leave to infuse for at least two weeks in a cool, dark place.

Strain the vinegar through cheesecloth or a fine-mesh strainer into a bowl or jug. Discard the herbs and peel. You will be surprised how good it smells!

The next step is to dilute the potent vinegar slightly by adding the water. The suggested ratio is 1:1.

Pour the mixture into a clean spray nozzle bottle/bottles.

Every time you use this herbal vinegar to clean your house, say: "I invite more love and light into my home. My home is surrounded by an aura of love."

The Ancient Greeks used oregano as an antidote to poisons. The Romans loved the taste of oregano so much that they used it to flavor everything, including wine. In the Middle Ages, oregano was used to treat indigestion, and raw leaves were chewed for oral hygiene.

PEONY SCRUB FOR COMPASSION

The peony is a symbol of compassion, love, and romance. And compassion is one of those treasures that we like to give to people around us, to strangers on the streets, and to our loved ones—but not to ourselves. Sometimes we dismiss the hardships of our own journey, and peony is one of those mystical flowers that can help you change that.

If you are lucky enough to find peonies during their short blooming period, preserve them in this salty body scrub. Let it be a reminder to show compassion for yourself. And to have a romance with yourself!

There is no other flower quite like the peony. The delicacy, the intoxicating aroma, the dreamy colors. They only bloom for a short period of time—a week if you are lucky—serving as a reminder to live life to the fullest, to be in the present moment, to seize the day and take advantage of opportunities when they come our way.

Ingredients:
handful of fresh peony petals
½ cup (120 g) fine sea salt
a few drops of your favorite essential oil
(rose goes well with peony)
2 tbsp apricot kernel oil, or any other light
oil of your choice

Equipment:
8 oz (225 ml) glass jar with lid

Directions:
In a food processor, blitz the peony petals and salt. The peony flowers will turn the mixture a wonderful pink color (make sure the flowers are completely dry before starting).

Spread the mixture in a single layer on a baking sheet covered with parchment paper to air-dry for a day or two. Stir a few times each day.

When the mixture is dry, add the oils and give everything a good stir.

Store in a jar with a tight lid in a cool place and out of direct sunlight.

Apply the scrub to damp skin and repeat the words: "I give myself the attention I deserve and need. I accept and love myself. I treat myself in the same way I would like others to treat me."

Rinse the scrub off with warm water.

When handling the scrub, make sure to use a spoon so that no water gets in the jar. This will ensure that the scrub stays fresh for several months.

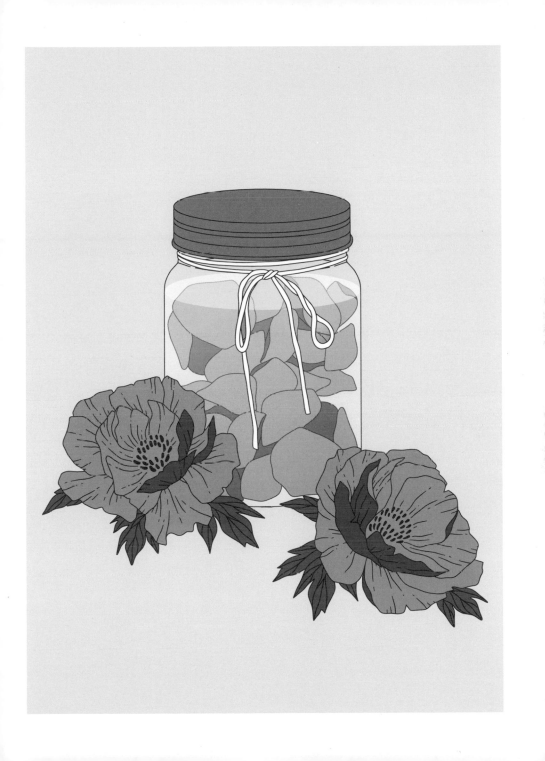

MYSTICAL RESINS TO CLEANSE AND BANISH

Just like vinegar and oregano, tree resin is a great help in removing stagnant and negative energy and creating a loving presence. There is a long history of using tree resin in ceremonies and divination practices all around the world—particularly frankincense and myrrh. Frankincense comes from the trunk of the Boswellia tree, while myrrh comes from an Arabian tree known as *Balsamodendron myrrha*, and their use in medicine, skincare, and cosmetics dates all the way back to Ancient Egypt.

But what intrigues me most is that they were also used to clear negativity, pessimism, and illusions that stand in the way of seeing the truth and fully enjoying life. It was believed that these resins had the power to enhance intuition and clairvoyance, and attract love. No wonder frankincense was once worth more than gold!

If you ever want to transform and banish unwanted energy, cleanse and bless your home, and connect to your higher self, try making this herbal cleansing blend.

Ingredients:
handful of frankincense resin
handful of myrrh resin
1 tsp dried mugwort (optional)
1 tsp dried rose petals (optional)
1 tsp dried lavender (optional)

Equipment:
charcoal disc
resin burner or any heatproof plate or bowl
  (ceramic, stone, even a large seashell)

Directions:

Start by mixing together the ingredients of your choice in a bowl.

Light the charcoal disc. It's best to hold the charcoal with tongs if you can. If not, hold it by one edge and light the other side. Place the charcoal on the burner.

Set a small amount of the blend in the indentation on top of the disc and let the smoke appear.

Slowly move around your home, allowing the smoke to cleanse and banish negativity. As you do so, think or speak out loud about all the things you want to clear your space of; what energies to transform: "I am cleansing my space from all the doubt, I am inviting more optimism and zest for life, I am banishing fear from my life and welcoming love instead, I am burning all the thoughts that caused me pain." Take as much time as you need.

Once finished, pour water on the charcoal and make sure it's completely extinguished. The remaining frankincense and myrrh blend will keep for years, stored in an airtight container away from moisture.

Some call resin "the blood" of the tree, some "the tears." But there is no question that resin plays an important part in the livelihood of the tree—it heals wounds, helps repair any damage, and protects against infection.

CRANBERRY FACIAL TONER
FOR MIRROR WORK

Whenever my teenage skin broke out in pimples, my mom would make a cranberry toner for me, squeezing the precious vitamins from the berries. I used it all through high school—I think the combination of my mother's loving words and the magic of cranberry helped to clear my skin. Now, any time my skin flares up, I make myself this cranberry toner, look in the mirror, and tell my skin how much I love her, how beautiful she is, and how no amount of pimples or blemishes can change that. It works every time!

Cranberries are one of the oldest superfoods—high in antioxidants and vitamin C. In Siberia, every fall my parents and I would visit the Narnia-like forest and gather cranberries. We would freeze the fresh berries and use them in winter for cold remedies, making jelly, jam, and tea with them. So many delicious treats!

Ingredients:
½ cup (120 ml) witch hazel
⅛ cup (30 ml) fresh cranberry juice
  (frozen berries work just as well as fresh)
⅛ cup (30 ml) rose water (optional)

Equipment:
4 oz (115 ml) glass jar with lid/spray bottle

Directions:
Combine all the ingredients in the jar of your choice and shake well.

Gently apply the toner with a cotton pad. As you do so, look in the mirror and tell your skin how much you love her, how much you appreciate her for protecting you every day, how it is ok to get irritated sometimes.

Store the toner in the fridge and use within 2–3 days.

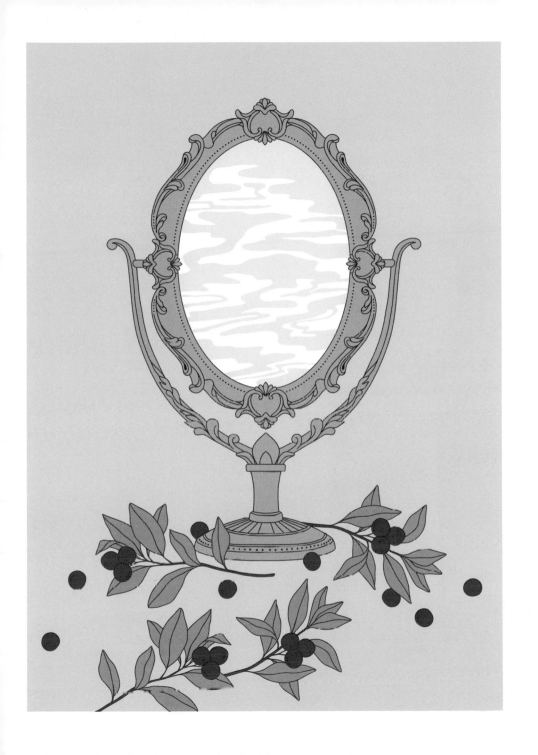

CHOCOLATE LIP BALM FOR DESIRE AND INNER-FIRE

If you have ever encountered cacao fruit in real life, you will know how intoxicating, delicious, tempting, moist, and just out of this world it is! Cacao is a sacred and nurturing plant, which has been around for thousands of years. Its aroma wraps you in a blanket of love, reminding you of your divine nature. Cacao is more than chocolate; it has the power to ignite the fire within you and burn away all that no longer serves you. It wakes up your emotional body, your feminine side, and serves as a reminder of how important it is to treat and spoil yourself, and to enjoy the sweetness of life, without feeling guilty.

Any time you need a reminder of your divine nature, or you want to awaken that fire and desire for life, sit with the medicine of cacao. Make yourself a hot cup of cacao and add a spoonful to your bath. Or try making this lip balm and carry it in your purse for an instant dose of love and desire.

Ingredients:
¼ cup (35 g) beeswax pellets
1 ½ tbsp coconut oil
a few drops of vitamin E oil
½ tbsp cacao powder or cocoa powder
2 tbsp virgin olive oil

Equipment:
heatproof bowl (glass or ceramic)
  or a canning jar
lip balm tubes
small funnel

Directions:

Combine the beeswax pellets, coconut oil, and vitamin E oil in the heatproof bowl. At the same time, put about 1 inch (2.5 cm) water into a saucepan over a low heat and place the bowl in the saucepan to create a double boiler. Stir constantly until all the ingredients have melted.

While the beeswax and oils are melting, whisk the cacao powder and olive oil together in a small bowl to combine. Cacao powder can be hard to incorporate sometimes, so make sure to break up all the lumps and keep mixing until smooth.

Once the beeswax and oils have completely melted, add the cacao powder mixture and stir well to combine.

While warm, pour the chocolate mixture into the tubes. Carefully fill one tube at a time using a small funnel. The chocolate balm will start to set as it cools down, so you need to work fast. Leave to cool for an hour or so before putting the caps on the tubes.

What's the difference between cocoa and cacao?
Both start out as beans from the cacao plant. After harvest, the beans are fermented to develop flavor and texture. Cacao powder is made from fermented beans that have not been roasted. They are processed at low temperatures then milled into a powder that's bitter in taste and higher in nutritional content. Cocoa powder is made from fermented beans that have been roasted, then processed at a much higher temperature. The result is a less bitter, slightly darker powder that has lost some of its nutritional value.

ENCYCLOPEDIA OF INGREDIENTS

EDIBLE FLOWERS

 Blue butterfly pea—to bring inspiration; to enhance psychic abilities

 Blue lotus—to enhance psychic abilities; to protect; to heal

 Calendula—to bring peace and joy; to heal; to make dreams come true; to gain strength

 California poppy—to ignite the inner-light; to be more open to new opportunities; to fear less

 Chamomile—to attract luck; to attract financial abundance; to enjoy a restful night's sleep; to ease anxiety

 Cornflower—to bring joy and enthusiasm for life; to bring love

 Cosmos—to bring harmony and love

 Daisy—to heal and nurture; to bring love

Dandelion—to bring light, love, and joy after difficult times

 Jasmine—to increase psychic abilities; to attract a lover

 Dianthus—to ground; to get in touch with your true self

 Lavender—to ease anxiety; to promote a good night's sleep; to welcome peace and harmony; to let go

 Echinacea—to heal; to gain strength; to protect

 Lilac—to gain wisdom; to find inspiration; to start anew

 Elderflower—to heal the physical and emotional body; to break a hex or negative thought pattern

 Magnolia—to celebrate spring; to ignite the life force; to welcome love into your heart

 Forget-me-not—to never forget how beautiful life is

 Nasturtium—to help balance emotions and rational thinking; to manifest

 Hibiscus—to connect to divine wisdom and consciousness; to attract love; to banish bad dreams

 Pansy—to love unconditionally; to attract love in all her forms; to improve relationships

Passionflower—to attract new people into your life; to bring peace; to reduce stress

 Sunflower—to bring energy; to restore power; to gain confidence and wisdom; to bring good memories back

 Peony—to be more compassionate; to live life to the fullest; to bring good fortune; to attract love

 Wild violet—to inspire and ignite the soul; to promote peace; to calm the nerves; to draw prophetic dreams and visions

 Red clover—to attract prosperity and good fortune

 Zinnia—to enjoy and love life just as it comes

 Rose—to promote love; to heal wounded love; to show love; to remind you that life is full of beauty

When working with fresh flowers, rinse them in cold water and allow to dry on a paper towel before using them in the recipes.

HERBS, SPICES, ROOTS, BARK

 Aloe vera—to regenerate and heal; to attract luck; to protect

 Borage—to help fight indecisiveness and doubt; to bring determination, courage, and self-confidence; to strengthen character; to increase psychic abilities

 Arnica—to nurture and protect

 Cayenne pepper—to repel negativity and unwanted energy

 Ashwagandha—to ease anxiety and stress; to promote peaceful and restful sleep

 Cedar—to gain confidence; to gain strength; to find power

 Basil—to attract wealth; to attract love; to protect

 Chive blossom—to have good times; to break negative habits

 Bay leaf—to make wishes come true; to see prophetic dreams; to alchemize desires; to purify; to remove obstacles; to bring success and good fortune

 Cinnamon—to see things as they truly are; to cleanse; to purify; to attract luck; to bring passion

 Bergamot—to promote self-acceptance and self-love; to bring more magic and love

 Clove—to attract luck; to gain clarity; to protect

133

Eucalyptus—to alleviate stress; to relax; to heal; to sharpen thought

 Mint—to bring back happy memories; to forget the past; to start afresh; to improve communication skills; to draw customers to a business

 Garlic—to heal and nourish; to banish evil spirits, envy, and jealousy

 Mugwort—to cleanse; to empower; to remember your powers and abilities

 Ginger—to increase personal power; to ignite the inner fire; to strengthen health; to forgive; to heal

 Nettle—to shift and transform your thoughts; to nurture the soul and heal the body; to remove jealous/envious thoughts; to protect; to strengthen your will

 Horsetail—to protect; to heal and repair

 Nutmeg—to attract good luck; to protect; to attract wealth; to break a hex

 Lemon balm—to heal your aching heart; to forgive; to rest; to ease anxiety; to let go

 Oregano—to cleanse; to infuse with an aura of love; to improve communication skills; to travel safely

 Marshmallow— to comfort

 Plantain weed—to release stagnant or negative feelings

Rosemary—to cleanse and purify your energy and space; to protect from negativity; to spark inspiration; to improve memory and concentration

 Turmeric—to brighten the day; to restore balance; to attract abundance

 Sage—to remove negative energy; to let go; to heal; to inspire; to boost creativity

 Vanilla—to restore any kind of relationship; to bring back love; to strengthen mental abilities

 Thyme—to feel courageous and brave; to protect and be protected; to attract abundance; to ward off nightmares; to ensure restful sleep

 Yarrow—to banish melancholy; to ground you; to gain a sense of control of your life

 Tulsi (holy basil)—to nourish the soul; to embody the Divine

BERRIES AND FRUITS

Cranberry—to protect oneself; to envision

Raspberries—to heal relationships; to attract happiness; to lift a mood; to energize; to promote self-love; to reduce anxiety; to bring light

Lemon—to bring back joy and happiness; to generate new ideas; to boost brain activity; to uplift; to energize; to remove unwanted energy; to bring light

Strawberries—to attract success; to attract good fortune; to connect to your inner goddess

Pomegranate—to embrace your dualities; to promote self-love; to use in divination rituals; to attract wealth; to increase fertility

CRYSTALS

Amethyst—to restore balance; to ground

Black tourmaline—to ground; to protect your aura

WITCHY PANTRY

 Candle—to cast magic

 Milk (any kind)—to heal; to soothe; to love; to experience hidden feelings so you can finally let them go

 Cacao— to awaken the inner fire and desire for life; to celebrate; to honor; to connect with divine wisdom

 Myrrh—to cleanse; to purify; to manifest; to protect from negative energies

 Frankincense—to cleanse, purify, and protect

 Oats—to cleanse; to bring clarity; to remove excess

 Green tea—to nurture; to protect; to forgive

 Salt—to cleanse and purify; to bring clarity; to remove excess

 Honey—to make wishes come true; to sweeten your path; to invoke the Goddess; to promote heart healing; to bring joy and laughter

CONCLUSION

Thank you, dear reader, for picking up this book and allowing me to share this magic with you. I hope it has inspired you to get your hands dirty—in the kitchen or in your garden—to admire every single flower, to pick your thoughts just like you pick your clothes (with intention), to speak to yourself with compassion and kindness and, most importantly, to love. We are multidimensional beings experiencing this life on Earth, and what a true gift it is to be alive and to love. Keep shining your light and loving yourself, unapologetically and fully.

FURTHER READING

Rosemary Gladstar's Medicinal Herbs: A Beginner's Guide: 33 Healing Herbs to Know, Grow, and Use, by Rosemary Gladstar (Storey Publishing, 2012)

Ritual Baths: Be Your Own Healer, by Deborah Hanekamp (Morrow Gift, 2020)

Inner Witch: A Modern Guide to the Ancient Craft, by Gabriela Herstik (TarcherPerigee, 2018)

The Green Witch: Your Complete Guide to the Natural Magic of Herbs, Flowers, Essential Oils, and More, by Arin Murphy-Hiscock (Adams Media, 2017)

Edible Flowers: How, Why and When We Eat Flowers, by Monica Nelson (The Monacelli Press, 2021)

ABOUT COSMIC VALERIA

Cosmic Valeria is a modern witch, herbalist, artist, and writer. She helps women to blend self-care and magic, reconnect with the energy of the moon, and celebrate the Divine Feminine that lives in all of us.

Born and raised in Siberia, Russia, she currently lives in the woods of Virginia, USA, with her partner and two cats.

Find more witchy inspiration at:

@cosmicvaleria

cosmicvaleria.com

INDEX

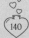

First published in 2023 by Leaping Hare Press
an imprint of The Quarto Group.
1 Triptych Place
London, SE1 9SH
United Kingdom
T (0)20 7700 6700
www.Quarto.com

A catalog record for this book is available
from the British Library.

ISBN 978-0-7112-8105-9
Ebook ISBN 9/8-0-7112-8106-6

10 9 8 7 6 5 4 3 2 1

Commissioning editor Chloe Murphy
Cover & interior illustrations by
Marie-Noël Dumont
Design by Nikki Ellis

Printed in China

The information in this book is for informational
purposes only and should not be treated as a
substitute for professional counselling, medical
advice or any medication or other treatment
prescribed by a medical practitioner; always
consult a medical professional. Any use of
the information in this book is at the reader's
discretion and risk. The author and publisher
make no representations or warranties with
respect to the accuracy, completeness or
fitness for a particular purpose of the contents
of this book and exclude all liability to the
extent permitted by law for any errors and
omissions and for any injury, loss, damage
or expense suffered by anyone arising out
of the use, or misuse, of the information in
this book, or any failure to take professional
medical advice.

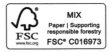